Iron Disorders

Editors

MATTHEW M. HEENEY
ALAN R. COHEN

HEMATOLOGY/ONCOLOGY CLINICS OF NORTH AMERICA

www.hemonc.theclinics.com

Consulting Editors
GEORGE P. CANELLOS
H. FRANKLIN BUNN

August 2014 • Volume 28 • Number 4

ELSEVIER

1600 John F. Kennedy Boulevard ● Suite 1800 ● Philadelphia, Pennsylvania, 19103-2899

http://www.theclinics.com

HEMATOLOGY/ONCOLOGY CLINICS OF NORTH AMERICA Volume 28, Number 4
August 2014 ISSN 0889-8588, ISBN 13: 978-0-323-29922-0

Editor: Jessica McCool
Developmental Editor: Donald Mumford

Hematology/Oncology Clinics (ISSN 0889-8588) is published bimonthly by Elsevier Inc., 360 Park Avenue South, New York, NY 10010-1710. Months of issue are February, April, June, August, October, and December. Business and Editorial Offices: 1600 John F. Kennedy Blvd., Ste. 1800, Philadelphia, PA 19103—2899. Customer Service Office: 3251 Riverport Lane, Maryland Heights, MO 63043. Periodicals postage paid at New York, NY and at additional mailing offices. Subscription prices are $385.00 per year (domestic individuals), $633.00 per year (domestic institutions), $190.00 per year (domestic students/residents), $440.00 per year (Canadian individuals), $783.00 per year (Canadian institutions) $520.00 per year (international individuals), $783.00 per year (international institutions), and $255.00 per year (international and Canadian students/residents). International air speed delivery is included in all *Clinics* subscription prices. All prices are subject to change without notice. **POSTMASTER:** Send address changes to *Hematology/Oncology Clinics of North America*, Elsevier Health Sciences Division, Subscription Customer Service, 3251 Riverport Lane, Maryland Heights, MO 63043. Customer Service (orders, claims, online, change of address): Elsevier Health Sciences Division, Subscription Customer Service, 3251 Riverport Lane, Maryland Heights, MO 63043. Tel: 1-800-654-2452 (U.S. and Canada); 314-447-8871 (outside U.S. and Canada). Fax: 314-447-8029. E-mail: journalscustomerservice-usa@elsevier.com (for print support); journalsonlinesupport-usa@elsevier.com (for online support).

Reprints. For copies of 100 or more, of articles in this publication, please contact the Commercial Reprints Department, Elsevier Inc., 360 Park Avenue South, New York, New York 10010-1710; Tel.: 212-633-3874, Fax: 212-633-3820, E-mail: reprints@elsevier.com.

Hematology/Oncology Clinics of North America is covered in *MEDLINE/PubMed (Index Medicus), EMBASE/ Excerpta Medica, and BIOSIS.*

Contributors

CONSULTING EDITORS

GEORGE P. CANELLOS, MD
William Rosenberg Professor of Medicine; Department of Medical Oncology, Dana-Farber Cancer Institute, Boston, Massachusetts

H. FRANKLIN BUNN, MD
Professor of Medicine; Division of Hematology, Brigham and Women's Hospital, Harvard Medical School, Boston, Massachusetts

EDITORS

MATTHEW M. HEENEY, MD
Assistant Professor of Pediatrics, Harvard Medical School; Associate Chief, Hematology, Division of Hematology/Oncology, Boston Children's Hospital, Boston, Massachusetts

ALAN R. COHEN, MD
Professor of Pediatrics, The Perelman School of Medicine at the University of Pennsylvania; Emeritus Chair of Pediatrics, and Physician-in-Chief, The Children's Hospital of Philadelphia, Philadelphia, Pennsylvania

AUTHORS

EDOUARD BARDOU-JACQUET, MD, PhD
CHU Rennes, French Reference Center for Rare Iron Overload Diseases of Genetic Origin; INSERM, UMR 991; Service des Maladies du Foie, CHU Rennes, Rennes, France

CATERINA BORGNA-PIGNATTI, MD
Chair of Pediatrics, Department of Medical Sciences, University of Ferrara, Ferrara, Italy

SYLVIA S. BOTTOMLEY, MD
Professor Emerita, Department of Medicine, University of Oklahoma College of Medicine, Oklahoma City, Oklahoma

PIERRE BRISSOT, MD, PhD
CHU Rennes, French Reference Center for Rare Iron Overload Diseases of Genetic Origin; INSERM, UMR 991; Service des Maladies du Foie, CHU Rennes, Rennes, France

GEORGE R. BUCHANAN, MD
Professor of Pediatrics, Pediatric Hematology-Oncology, University of Texas Southwestern Medical Center, Dallas, Texas

KARIN E. FINBERG, MD, PhD
Assistant Professor of Pathology, Department of Pathology, Yale School of Medicine, New Haven, Connecticut

MARK D. FLEMING, MD, DPhil
Pathologist-in-Chief; S. Burt Wolbach Professor of Pathology, Department of Pathology, Boston Children's Hospital, Harvard Medical School, Boston, Massachusetts

TOMAS GANZ, MD, PhD
Professor of Medicine and Pathology, Departments of Medicine and Pathology, David Geffen School of Medicine at University of California, Los Angeles, Los Angeles, California

MACIEJ GARBOWSKI, MD
Department of Haematology, University College London, London, United Kingdom

MATTHEW M. HEENEY, MD
Assistant Professor of Pediatrics, Harvard Medical School; Associate Chief, Hematology, Division of Hematology/Oncology, Boston Children's Hospital, Boston, Massachusetts

MARIA MARSELLA, MD
Professor of Pediatrics, Department of Medical Sciences, University of Ferrara, Ferrara, Italy

ELIZABETA NEMETH, PhD
Professor of Medicine, Department of Medicine, David Geffen School of Medicine at University of California, Los Angeles, Los Angeles, California

JOHN B. PORTER, MD
Department of Haematology, University College London, London, United Kingdom

JACQUELYN M. POWERS, MD
Fellow, Pediatric Hematology-Oncology, University of Texas Southwestern Medical Center, Dallas, Texas

JOHN C. WOOD, MD, PhD
Professor of Pediatrics and Radiology; Director of Cardiovascular MRI, Department of Pediatrics and Radiology, Children's Hospital, Los Angeles, Keck School of Medicine, University of Southern California, Los Angeles, California

Contents

The management and understanding of hereditary hemochromatosis have evolved with recent advances in iron biology and the associated discovery of numerous genes involved in iron metabolism. *HFE*-related (type 1) hemochromatosis remains the most frequent form, characterized by C282Y mutation homozygosity. Rare forms of hereditary hemochromatosis include type 2 (A and B, juvenile hemochromatosis caused by *HJV* and *HAMP* mutation), type 3 (related to *TFR2* mutation), and type 4 (A and B, ferroportin disease). The diagnostic evaluation relies on comprehension of the involved pathophysiologic defect, and careful characterization of the phenotype, which gives clues to guide appropriate genetic testing.

Iron deficiency anemia is a common global problem whose etiology is typically attributed to inadequate dietary intake and/or chronic blood loss. However, in several kindreds multiple family members are affected with iron deficiency anemia that is unresponsive to oral iron supplementation and only partially responsive to parenteral iron therapy. The discovery that many of these cases harbor mutations in the *TMPRSS6* gene led to the recognition that they represent a single clinical entity: iron-refractory iron deficiency anemia (IRIDA). This article reviews clinical features of IRIDA, recent genetic studies, and insights this disorder provides into the regulation of systemic iron homeostasis.

Sideroblastic anemias (SAs) may be acquired or congenital and share the features of disrupted utilization of iron in the erythroblast, ineffective erythropoiesis, and variable systemic iron overload. Congenital forms can have associated syndromic features or be nonsyndromic, and many of them have mutations in genes encoding proteins involved in heme biosynthesis, iron-sulfur cluster biogenesis, or mitochondrial protein synthesis. The mechanism(s) for the acquired clonal SA is undefined and is under intense study. Precise diagnosis of these disorders rests on careful clinical and laboratory evaluation, including molecular analysis. Supportive treatments usually provide for a favorable prognosis and often for normal survival.

Acquired Iron Disorders

Anemia of inflammation (AI, also called anemia of chronic disease) is a common, typically normocytic, normochromic anemia that is caused by an underlying inflammatory disease. It is diagnosed when serum iron concentrations are low despite adequate iron stores, as evidenced by serum ferritin that is not low. In the setting of inflammation, it may be difficult to differentiate AI from iron deficiency anemia, and the 2 conditions may co-exist. Treatment should focus on the underlying disease. Recent advances in molecular understanding of AI are stimulating the development of new pathophysiologically targeted experimental therapies.

The pathophysiologic consequences of transfusional iron overload (TIO) as well as the benefits of iron chelation therapy are best described in thalassemia major, although TIO is increasingly seen in other clinical settings. These consequences broadly reflect the levels and distribution of excess storage iron in the heart, endocrine tissues, and liver. TIO also increases the risk of infection, due to increased availability of labile iron to microorganisms. The authors suggest that extrahepatic iron distribution, and hence toxicity, is influenced by balance between generation of nontransferrin-bound iron from red cell catabolism and the utilization of transferrin iron by the erythron.

 Video demonstrating a schedule of administration of iron chelators accompanies this article

Iron overload is an inevitable consequence of blood transfusions and is often accompanied by increased iron absorption from the gut. Chelation therapy is necessary to prevent the consequences of hemosiderosis. Three chelators, deferoxamine, deferiprone, and deferasirox, are presently available and a fourth is undergoing clinical trials. The efficacy of all 3 available chelators has been demonstrated. Also, many studies have shown the efficacy of the combination of deferoxamine plus deferiprone as an intensive treatment of severe iron overload. Alternating chelators can reduce adverse effects and improve compliance. Adherence to therapy is crucial for good results.

Iron-Related Monitoring and Therapy

Iron deficiency anemia (IDA) is a common hematologic condition, affecting a substantial proportion of the world's women and young children. Optimal management of IDA requires an accurate diagnosis, identification and correction of the underlying cause, provision of medicinal iron therapy, and confirmation of treatment success. There are limited data to support current treatment approaches regarding oral iron preparation, dosing, monitoring, and duration of therapy. New intravenous iron agents have improved safety profiles, which may foster their increased utilization in the treatment of patients with IDA. Clinical trials focused on improving current treatment standards for IDA are sorely needed.

John C. Wood

Treatment of iron overload requires robust estimates of total-body iron burden and its response to iron chelation therapy. Compliance with chelation therapy varies considerably among patients, and individual reporting is notoriously unreliable. Even with perfect compliance, intersubject variability in chelator effectiveness is extremely high, necessitating reliable iron estimates to guide dose titration. In addition, each chelator has a unique profile with respect to clearing iron stores from different organs. This article presents the tools available to clinicians to monitor their patients, focusing on noninvasive magnetic resonance imaging methods because they have become the de facto standard of care.

HEMATOLOGY/ONCOLOGY
CLINICS OF NORTH AMERICA

VISIT THE CLINICS ONLINE!
Access your subscription at:
www.theclinics.com

NOW AVAILABLE FOR YOUR iPhone and iPad

Preface

Iron Disorders

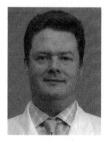 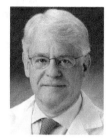

Matthew M. Heeney, MD   Alan R. Cohen, MD
Editors

Ferric (Fe^{+3}) iron is ubiquitous in the earth's environment and an essential metal in the biological processes of many organisms. In mammals, the major role of iron is to provide a binding site for oxygen in the heme moiety of hemoglobin. However, iron also plays a central role in the reduction/oxidation reactions performed by numerous cytochromes, peroxidases, ribonucleotide reductases, and catalases. This essential reactivity also has the potential to do great damage to macromolecular cellular components and tissues if iron is not chaperoned by iron-binding proteins.

Recent discoveries of mutations in genes leading to inherited diseases of iron overload and iron deficiency have advanced the understanding of iron homeostasis in humans. Articles from Bardou-Jacquet and Brissot, and Heeney and Finberg provide strategies for diagnosis and management of inherited iron overload and inherited iron deficiency, respectively. Inherited sideroblastic anemias are a heterogeneous group of diseases whose phenotype includes the accumulation of mitochondrial iron related to defective heme biosynthesis, iron-sulfur cluster biogenesis, or mitochondrial protein synthesis. In their article, Bottomley and Fleming summarize the heterogeneous phenotypes and the known mutations that explain the disorders in approximately two-thirds of the patients.

Of course, not all iron-related disease is congenital. Acquired iron deficiency is estimated to affect over one billion persons and is the most common cause of the nutritional anemias. Powers and Buchanan review iron deficiency and the dearth of well-designed clinical trials for its treatment and touch on some of the newer parenteral iron therapies. The discovery of hepcidin as the central regulator of iron metabolism has led to intense research into the regulation of hepcidin itself. The effect of chronic inflammation on iron homeostasis and the anemia of chronic inflammation is expertly reviewed by Nemeth and Ganz. The regulatory effect of iron stores on hepcidin is trumped by the ineffective erythropoiesis of the thalassemia syndromes, yet the exact mechanism is unclear. The pathophysiology of acquired transfusional iron overload and the central role of "unchaperoned" iron is reviewed by Porter and Garbowski.

Hematol Oncol Clin N Am 28 (2014) ix–x
http://dx.doi.org/10.1016/j.hoc.2014.05.001
0889-8588/14/$ – see front matter © 2014 Elsevier Inc. All rights reserved.

hemonc.theclinics.com

Marsella and Borgna-Pignatti then summarize the current use of iron chelation therapy in thalassemia major and sickle cell disease.

The monitoring of iron overload is addressed in the final article. Wood reviews the history of methods of iron assessment and focuses on the use of magnetic resonance as the de facto gold standard for noninvasive multiorgan iron quantification.

Together, these articles provide a detailed view of the remarkable advances in our understanding of the role of iron in human health and disease, and we are very grateful to the authors for their renowned work in this field and their thoughtful contributions to this issue.

Matthew M. Heeney, MD
Division of Hematology/Oncology
Boston Children's Hospital
300 Longwood Avenue
Boston, MA 02115, USA

Alan R. Cohen, MD
The Children's Hospital of Philadelphia
34th Street and Civic Center Boulevard
Philadelphia, PA 19104, USA

E-mail addresses:
Matthew.Heeney@childrens.harvard.edu (M.M. Heeney)
cohen@email.chop.edu (A.R. Cohen)

Diagnostic Evaluation of Hereditary Hemochromatosis (HFE and Non-HFE)

Edouard Bardou-Jacquet, MD, PhD[a,b,c,*], Pierre Brissot, MD, PhD[a,b,c]

KEYWORDS

- Hemochromatosis • Hepcidin • HFE • TFR2 • Hemojuvelin • Ferroportin
- Phlebotomy

KEY POINTS

- Hereditary hemochromatosis can damage liver, heart, pancreas, endocrine glands, bones, and joints. However clinical expression spans from a few biologic anomalies to full-blown multiorgan involvement.
- Hereditary hemochromatosis is mainly related to inappropriately deficient hepcidin secretion related to mutations in genes involved in hepcidin regulation.
- Ferroportin disease is associated with normal hepcidin secretion, but mutations in ferroportin induce loss of iron export function or resistance to hepcidin regulation.
- *HFE*-related hemochromatosis is the most frequent form in the white population. Genetic testing for rare forms of hereditary hemochromatosis must be guided by the clinical phenotype.

INTRODUCTION

To efficiently assess patients with suspected hereditary hemochromatosis, clinicians must understand the normal physiology of iron metabolism and the pathophysiologic mechanisms leading to iron overload.

Iron Metabolism

Iron absorption and export
Iron absorption occurs in the proximal duodenum. Nonheme iron is transported across the luminal membrane of the duodenal enterocyte into the cytoplasm by divalent metal

[a] CHU Rennes, French Reference Center for Rare Iron Overload Diseases of Genetic Origin, 2 rue Henri le guilloux, F-35033 Rennes, France; [b] INSERM, UMR 991, 2 rue Henri le guilloux, F-35000 Rennes, France; [c] CHU Rennes, Liver disease department, 2 rue Henri le guilloux, F-35033 Rennes, France
* Corresponding author. CHU Rennes, French Reference Center for Rare Iron Overload Diseases of Genetic Origin, 2 rue Henri le guilloux, F-35033 Rennes, France.
E-mail address: edouard.bardou-jacquet@chu-rennes.fr

Hematol Oncol Clin N Am 28 (2014) 625–635
http://dx.doi.org/10.1016/j.hoc.2014.04.006
0889-8588/14/$ – see front matter © 2014 Elsevier Inc. All rights reserved.

transporter 1.[1] Transport of heme iron into the enterocyte membrane is performed by a pathway that remains controversial.

Ferroportin (SLCA40A1)[2] is located at the basolateral membrane of the enterocyte and at the membrane of macrophages. It is the only known cellular iron exporter, allowing iron egress from the cytoplasm into the bloodstream.

Hepcidin

Hepcidin (HAMP)[3] is synthesized primarily by hepatocytes, but is also produced at lower levels by adipocytes and macrophages. This small peptide, initially identified as an anti-microbial peptide, was later shown to be the key hormone regulator of iron metabolism.[4,5]

Hepcidin regulates iron availability through the modulation of iron export by ferroportin: hepcidin binds to ferroportin at the membrane of enterocytes or macrophages, and causes subsequent ferroportin endocytosis and degradation, thus impairing iron export.[6]

Hepcidin regulation

Because of its central role in iron metabolism, hepcidin is tightly regulated by several pathways including inflammation, erythropoiesis, and body iron stores. The regulation of hepcidin according to body iron stores involves distinct pathways for long- and short-term regulation. Basal expression is regulated through a bone morphogenetic protein/ Son of Mother Against Decapentaplegic (SMAD) pathway. Bone morphogenetic protein 6 plays a major role in association with its coreceptor hemojuvelin (HJV),[7] and is also involved in the response of hepcidin expression to iron stores over the long term.

Regarding the short-term regulation, it is proposed to be mediated through serum transferrin saturation.[8] Although the molecular mechanisms remain debated, it is proposed that HFE, TFR1, TFR2, and HJV form an iron-sensing complex at the hepatocyte membrane, with subsequent regulation of hepcidin expression.

Iron Overload

Iron overload in hereditary hemochromatosis occurs through two main distinct mechanisms.

Hepcidin deficiency

Hepcidin deficiency is the key mechanism of iron overload in HFE, HJV, HAMP, and TFR2 related hemochromatosis.[9] Mutations in these genes lead to defective or inappropriately low hepatic synthesis of hepcidin for the degree of iron burden. In HFE hemochromatosis it has been demonstrated that correction of liver hepcidin secretion normalized iron metabolism, confirming the predominant role of liver.[10]

Relative hepcidin deficiency leads to a sustained and unregulated activity of ferroportin with two consequences: increased duodenal iron absorption, and enhanced release of iron from reticuloendothelial macrophages into the bloodstream originating from erythrophagocytosis.

The overall result is increased plasma iron concentration and increased saturation of transferrin. If the capacity of transferrin is exceeded, an abnormal physiologic form of iron appears, called nontransferrin bound iron. Nontransferrin bound iron is rapidly taken up by the liver, pancreas, and heart, and leads to pathologic parenchymal iron deposition and organ dysfunction. Moreover, if transferrin saturation exceeds 75%, labile plasma iron appears, which has a high propensity for generating reactive oxygen species that can directly damage tissues.[11]

Ferroportin disease

There are two types of ferroportin disease that are distinguished by the molecular mechanism involved. Type A is characterized by a loss of ferroportin activity caused by mutations in the *SLC40A1* gene.[12] As a consequence of the functional deficiency, macrophage iron overload results from decreased iron export. The pathologic consequence is reticuloendothelial macrophage iron loading. Type B is characterized by mutations in ferroportin, which confer "resistance" to hepcidin.[13] Thus, despite an increased serum hepcidin level, ferroportin regulation is defective, resulting in constitutive ferroportin activity and a "functional" hepcidin deficiency, as in HFE hemochromatosis. The pathologic consequence is reticuloendothelial macrophage iron sparing and parenchymal iron loading in target organs.

Penetrance

Clinical expression in hereditary hemochromatosis is variable, especially regarding *HFE* hemochromatosis.[14] This variable phenotype makes it difficult to define hereditary hemochromatosis: does it correspond only to the identification of genetic mutations, to the association of biologic iron overload with genetic mutations, or only to iron-related clinical expression? Moreover, for the latter two conditions, the clinically significant level of iron overload remains to be determined.

HFE hemochromatosis is primarily associated with homozygosity for the C282Y *HFE* mutation. However, depending on the diagnostic criteria used, clinically significant iron overload is observed in only 5% to 75% of homozygotes patients.[14,15] A recent meta-analysis showed an overall penetrance of 13.5%,[16] and longitudinal studies showed iron overload in up to 50% of patients.

This variable penetrance is caused by numerous other acquired and genetic factors affecting iron metabolism regulation. Male sex[17] and alcohol consumption[18] increase the severity of iron overload, whereas obesity, through higher hepcidin expression, has been proposed to exert a protective effect.[19] Furthermore, the occurrence of mutations in other genes involved in iron metabolism has been showed to modify the iron burden; however, the search for other genetic factors has shown variable results.[20,21]

Because of the relatively few cases of type 2 and 3 hemochromatosis described, data regarding their penetrance and expression are scarce. If the penetrance is nearly complete, the severity of iron burden and age of presentation seems to be more variable than initially thought. This may be caused by the same reasons as seen in *HFE* hemochromatosis, but likely also related to the nature and consequences of the specific mutations involved.

Diagnostic Work-up

We must consider that hereditary hemochromatosis encompasses a wide continuum of hepcidin deficiency states, whose clinical expression varies according to the main genes involved and the subsequent impaired molecular mechanisms. Moreover, clinical expression can be further modified by other acquired and genetics factors.

Therefore, the diagnostic evaluation requires a careful characterization of the patient's phenotype, and an accurate assessment of iron overload and potential disease modifiers. Then, the phenotype guides the clinician through the appropriate genetic testing for determination of the genes and mutations involved.

PATIENT HISTORY

The patient history is a crucial element for accurate diagnosis, avoidance of being misled by confounding factors, and to optimize resource use. Regarding the laboratory evaluation, it should be emphasized that because of significant variability of biochemical iron parameters (transferrin saturation) related to diurnal variation and sensitivity to dietary iron, repeated early morning and fasting measurements should be performed.[22]

Family history is also a cornerstone of the diagnostic evaluation. Search for putative diagnosis of iron overload in relatives can suggest a dominant or recessive inheritance pattern and strengthen the need for genetic evaluation of an individual or family.

Careful search for possible causes of secondary iron overload (**Box 1**) and potential confounding factors or acquired modifiers of iron burden (**Box 2**) help the clinician in the assessment of iron overload.

PHYSICAL EXAMINATION

Clinical features of hereditary hemochromatosis are diverse and can be constitutional complaints, such as fatigue and mood disturbance, or related to organ toxicity and dysfunction, such as impotence, arthropathy, osteoporosis, dark skin, hepatomegaly, diabetes, and cardiomyopathy (cardiac failure or rhythm disturbance). However, the current major cause of referral is an elevated serum ferritin level, detected in the context of suspected iron overload, or as an incidental finding during routine check-up or evaluation for other suspected diseases.

Organs Involved in Hereditary Hemochromatosis

Liver disease

The liver is the main storage site for iron in normal physiology, and has a high affinity for nontransferrin bound iron. Liver iron concentration measured by liver biopsy is accepted as a surrogate marker of total body iron stores, although there are acknowledged problems with sampling variability. Oxidative stress and reactive oxygen species induced by iron overload and other possible comorbidities (eg, alcohol consumption) lead to hepatocellular necrosis, fibrosis, and eventually cirrhosis.

Liver-related mortality, especially caused by hepatocellular carcinoma, is the main cause of death of patients with *HFE* hemochromatosis, and is directly related to the degree of liver fibrosis.[23] Proper assessment of liver fibrosis is thus mandatory and can be performed by surrogate markers (biologic tests and/or scores[24–26]) or by liver biopsy. Significant fibrosis occurs only with significant iron overload and can thus be ruled out if serum ferritin is below 1000 μg/L and no other comorbidities are present.[26]

Bones and joints

Joint pain in hereditary hemochromatosis is similar to that of chondrocalcinosis or arthritis. Up to one-third of patients with *HFE* hemochromatosis can present with

---

Box 1
Causes of secondary iron overload

- Parenteral iron supplementation

    Ensure that the patient has not undergone prolonged iron supplementation, especially in a patient with chronic anemia or seeking enhanced sport performance.

- Oral iron supplementation

    Has been described as a potential cause of iron overload, but is controversial.

- Hematologic conditions

    Chronic or rare anemias can be associated with iron overload through repeated transfusions and/or hepcidin deficiency (ineffective erythropoiesis leads to inhibition of hepcidin expression) possibly through erythroferrone.[40]

- History of chemotherapy

    Growth factors or transfusions used in this context can also lead to iron overload.

Box 2
Cofounding factors and modifiers of iron burden

- Alcohol consumption

  Alcohol can induce ferritin synthesis, inhibits hepcidin synthesis, and causes liver damage, which may increase serum ferritin. Serum ferritin should be assessed after a period of abstinence.

- Metabolic syndrome

  Metabolic syndrome causes high serum ferritin without or with mild iron overload. Transferrin saturation is usually normal or slightly increased.

- Inflammation

  In the acute or chronic phase of inflammation, ferritin can be mobilized, leading to high serum ferritin without iron excess.

- Liver damage

  Hepatocyte injury can lead to release of intracellular ferritin into the bloodstream.

---

arthropathy.[14] The second and third metacarpophalangeal joints are the most frequently involved. Wrists, hips, and knees can also be involved, and require more frequent surgery than in the general population. The pathophysiology of joint disease is unclear and joint pain is often unresponsive to iron depletion treatment and can even worsen despite normalized iron burden. Hereditary hemochromatosis can be associated with osteoporosis (up to 25% of patients) with increased fracture risk.

Heart

Cardiac myocytes, like hepatocytes, have a high affinity for nontransferrin bound iron. In the heart, iron overload occurs mainly in ventricles where it induces fibrosis and alteration of myocardial fibers. The level of iron overload at which cardiac involvement is significant has not yet been clearly defined.[16]

As iron overload severity increases, diastolic dysfunction of the left ventricle occurs first, followed by impaired systolic dysfunction. Heart rhythm disorders can also occur. Cardiac echocardiography can detect early cardiac dysfunction, and cardiac iron overload can be assessed by magnetic resonance imaging (see article by Wood elsewhere in this issue). Iron depletion treatment has been shown to improve cardiac function.[27]

Pancreas

Although iron overload occurs mainly in the pancreatic acinar cells and not in β-islets, pancreatic endocrine dysfunction and diabetes are a well-described feature of hereditary hemochromatosis. However, pancreatic iron overload occurs only in severe forms of hereditary hemochromatosis and thus the prevalence of hemochromatosis-associated diabetes has decreased in recent years with earlier diagnosis.

Pituitary

Iron overload can involve the anterior pituitary and alter the gonadotropin pathway, leading to loss of libido, impotence, reduced testicular volume in males, and amenorrhea in females. However, this generally only occurs in cases of massive iron overload. If iron overload is very early, the patient can present with delayed pubertal development.

Clinical Presentation According the Type of Hereditary Hemochromatosis

Hepcidin deficiency

According to the genes involved and the subsequent affected mechanisms, pheno-type differs between types of hereditary hemochromatosis. Age of onset, severity of iron burden, and the type of organ involved therefore vary, making it difficult to describe "a classical pattern" of hereditary hemochromatosis that helps the clinician with the diagnosis work-up (**Table 1**).

Ferroportin disease

Ferroportin disease, consistent with its unique pathophysiology, presents as a different phenotype from hepcidin deficiency–related hereditary hemochromatosis (see **Table 1**). Type A and type B ferroportin are defined according to serum transferrin saturation: type A, loss of ferroportin activity → iron trapped in macrophages → serum transferrin saturation is normal or low; type B, ferroportin resistance to hepcidin → constitutive ferroportin activity and iron export → serum transferrin saturation is high. Actually, in the classical type A form, iron overload can be massive but the clin-ical consequences seem to be relatively low in the absence of cofactors, whereas in the rarer type B form, liver fibrosis can be present.[28]

TYPES OF HEREDITARY HEMOCHROMATOSIS AND GENETIC TESTING

Before initiating genetic testing, one must first rule out misleading causes of high serum ferritin (**Box 3**). Then, the body iron burden must be determined (see Wood article). Liver biopsy can be used to assess body iron burden, but is invasive and prone to sampling error if there is fibrosis/cirrhosis and heterogeneous iron deposition. Liver iron concentration determination by magnetic resonance imaging techniques is becoming the gold standard method and assessment of other organs.

The Different Types of Hereditary Hemochromatosis

Type 1 (HFE related) hemochromatosis

HFE-related hemochromatosis is the classical form of hereditary hemochromatosis. The *HFE* gene codes the MHC-like membrane protein HFE, whose definite role remains unclear.

The most common causative HFE mutation is the homozygous p.Cys282Tyr (C282Y) mutation.[29] The prevalence of this mutation is high in white populations (homozygotes, 3%–5%), but almost absent in nonwhite populations.[16]

Table 1
Different types of hereditary hemochromatosis according to the genes involved and their classical phenotypes

	Gene	Usual Age of Onset	Iron Burden	Liver	Bones and Joints	Heart	Pituitary
Type 1	HFE	~40–60	+/+++	++	++	+	+
Type 2A	HJV	~15	+++	+++	++	+++	++++
Type 2B	HAMP	~15	+++	+++	++	+++	++++
Type 3	TFR2	~30+	+++	+++	++	+	++
Type 4A	SLC40A1	Any	+/+++	?	–	–	–
Type 4B	SLC40A1	Any	+/+++	++	–	–	–

Age indicates usual age of onset. Iron burden indicates the usual severity of iron overload.

Box 3
Alternative causes of elevated serum ferritin

- Gaucher disease

    Anemia, thrombocytopenia, hepatosplenomegaly, and bone pains

- Macrophage activation syndrome

    Fever, splenomegaly, cytopenia, high serum triglycerides

- Hereditary hyperferritinemia cataract syndrome

    High serum ferritin with history of early cataract formation with dominant transmission, caused by mutations of the iron responsive element in the noncoding region of the mRNA of the L-ferritin gene

---

Other genotypes commonly included in HFE sequencing by clinical laboratories (eg, H63D and S65C) cannot explain overt iron overload and do not lead to clinically significant iron overload in the absence of comorbidities (alcoholism or metabolic syndrome).[30]

Compound heterozygosity (C282Y/H63D) may induce mild to moderate iron overload with increased transferrin saturation and serum ferritin. Compound heterozygote C282Y/H63D patients generally do not develop overt iron overload, but similarly not all patients with C282Y homozygosity develop iron overload (low penetrance), thus the clinical relevance of compound heterozygosity is still debated.[16]

Other rare (private) HFE mutations have been described associated with those frequent genotypes, thus explaining unusual cases of iron overload.[31]

Type 2 (HJV and HAMP related) hemochromatosis

Type 2A hemochromatosis is caused by mutations of the *HJV* gene[32] and type IIB is caused by mutations of the hepcidin (*HAMP*) gene[33] itself. Both are autosomal-recessive diseases. Patients usually present at an earlier age (<20 years old), and often with cardiac and central endocrine involvement (hypogonadotropic hypogonadism). Iron overload is massive and although liver fibrosis is frequent, cardiac and endocrine manifestations are predominant.

Type 3 (TFR2 related) hemochromatosis

Type III hemochromatosis is caused by mutations in the transferrin receptor 2 (*TFR2*) gene.[34] It can be considered an "intermediate" condition between juvenile and *HFE* hemochromatosis. Transmission is also autosomal-recessive.

The clinical picture of type 3 hemochromatosis is similar to that of *HFE* hemochromatosis, although patients are usually younger and iron overload more severe.[35] Cardiac and endocrine dysfunctions are less frequent than in juvenile hemochromatosis. Arthropathy is not uncommon.

Type 4 hemochromatosis: ferroportin disease

Mutations of the ferroportin (*SLC40A1*) gene lead to autosomal-dominant iron overload.[36] Type 4 hemochromatosis is more frequent than types 2 and 3 hemochromatosis and it has been reported in a wide range of populations. Ferroportin disease can be subdivided into two subtypes according to the molecular impact of the mutations.[37]

Type 4A ferroportin disease is caused by loss of the iron-export function.[12] The subsequent iron accumulation within macrophages accounts for the predominant spleen iron overload and the low biologic availability explaining normal (or low) transferrin saturation.

Type 4B ferroportin disease, which is rarer, is caused by resistance of ferroportin to hepcidin activity, resulting in an unregulated cellular iron egress.[38] The phenotypic picture is similar to that of *HFE* hemochromatosis with increased transferrin saturation, and hepatocyte iron deposition.

Other rare iron overload diseases
Mutations of the ceruloplasmin gene (hereditary aceruloplasminemia) either inhibit protein production or its ferroxidase activity. Iron overload is associated with anemia, neurologic symptoms, and diabetes.[39] Other rare entities present as anemia and iron overload syndromes: these include mutations of transferrin (atransferrinemia), divalent metal transporter 1, and congenital sideroblastic anemias (see article by Bottomley and Fleming elsewhere in this issue).

Genetic Testing

Identification of the genetic cause of primary iron overload is guided by the combination of patient's clinical and laboratory data that suggest the possible underlying pathophysiologic mechanism. This clinical guidance of the suspected underlying genetic cause facilitates a rational, step-wise evaluation. This efficient approach is warranted until next-generation sequencing is available, because most of the genetic studies are expensive and time consuming.

The decision tree toward genetic evaluation of patients with elevated ferritin is summarized in **Figs. 1** and **2**. Measurement of serum transferrin saturation is the pivotal first step.

Increased transferrin saturation
The most likely diagnosis in whites is *HFE* related (or type 1) hemochromatosis as confirmed by *HFE* C282Y homozygosity (see **Fig. 1**). If there is a family history of dominant transmission the patient should be evaluated for type 4B hemochromatosis ferroportin disease.

If the C282Y *HFE* mutation is absent, the next relevant information is the age of onset:

- Young patients (<20 years old) suggest type 2 hemochromatosis, either type 2A (HJV mutations) or type 2B (hepcidin mutation).

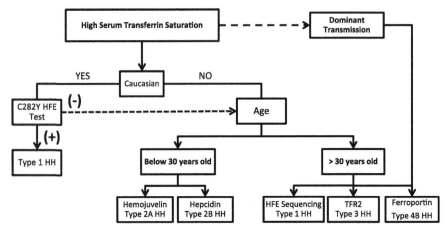

Fig. 1. Guide to genetic testing for hereditary hemochromatosis if transferrin saturation is high. HH, hereditary hemochromatosis.

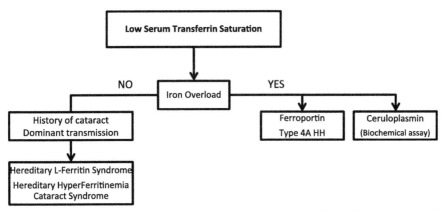

Fig. 2. Guide to genetic testing for hereditary hemochromatosis if transferrin saturation is low or normal. HH, hereditary hemochromatosis.

- Older patients suggest type 3 hemochromatosis (*TFR2*), type 4B ferroportin disease, or private mutations of the *HFE* gene. Private mutations require complete sequencing of the gene instead of the routine targeted *HFE* C282Y sequencing.
- However, juvenile onset of type 3 hemochromatosis and, conversely, late onset of type II hemochromatosis have been reported. Age is a clue for deciding which genetic test should be performed first.

Normal or low transferrin saturation

The most likely diagnosis is the classical form of ferroportin disease (type 4A hemochromatosis) (see **Fig. 2**). In this setting and if diabetes, anemia, and/or neurologic symptoms are present, hereditary aceruloplasminemia may be considered. Given its simplicity, plasma ceruloplasmin levels should be determined first. In this disorder, ceruloplasmin levels are typically undetectable, but in some cases ceruloplasmin is only significantly decreased.

SUMMARY

The diagnostic evaluation of hereditary hemochromatosis relies on proper clinical and laboratory evaluation of the patient, and on the understanding of the underlying pathophysiologic mechanisms. Recent improved understanding of normal iron metabolism has elucidated the pathophysiology of the different types of iron overload, allowing genetic diagnosis of most cases of hereditary hemochromatosis. In the next few years, the availability of "next-generation sequencing" will allow easier and faster access to genetic diagnosis of hereditary iron overload disorders.

REFERENCES

1. Gunshin H, Fujiwara Y, Custodio AO, et al. Slc11a2 is required for intestinal iron absorption and erythropoiesis but dispensable in placenta and liver. J Clin Invest 2005;115(5):1258–66.
2. Donovan A, Brownlie A, Zhou Y, et al. Positional cloning of zebrafish ferroportin1 identifies a conserved vertebrate iron exporter. Nature 2000;403(6771):776–81.
3. Park CH, Valore EV, Waring AJ, et al. Hepcidin, a urinary antimicrobial peptide synthesized in the liver. J Biol Chem 2001;276(11):7806–10.

4. Pigeon C, Ilyin G, Courselaud B, et al. A new mouse liver-specific gene, encoding a protein homologous to human antimicrobial peptide hepcidin, is overexpressed during iron overload. J Biol Chem 2001;276(11):7811–9.

5. Nicolas G, Bennoun M, Devaux I, et al. Lack of hepcidin gene expression and severe tissue iron overload in upstream stimulatory factor 2 (USF2) knockout mice. Proc Natl Acad Sci U S A 2001;98(15):8780–5.

6. Nemeth E, Tuttle MS, Powelson J, et al. Hepcidin regulates cellular iron efflux by binding to ferroportin and inducing its internalization. Science 2004;306(5704): 2090–3.

7. Meynard D, Kautz L, Darnaud V, et al. Lack of the bone morphogenetic protein BMP6 induces massive iron overload. Nat Genet 2009;41(4):478–81.

8. Goswami T, Andrews NC. Hereditary hemochromatosis protein, HFE, interaction with transferrin receptor 2 suggests a molecular mechanism for mammalian iron sensing. J Biol Chem 2006;281(39):28494–8.

9. Papanikolaou G, Tzilianos M, Christakis JI, et al. Hepcidin in iron overload disorders. Blood 2005;105(10):4103–5.

10. Bardou-Jacquet E, Philip J, Lorho R, et al. Liver transplantation normalizes serum hepcidin level and cures iron metabolism alterations in HFE hemochromatosis. Hepatology 2014;59(3):839–47.

11. Le Lan C, Loreal O, Cohen T, et al. Redox active plasma iron in C282Y/C282Y hemochromatosis. Blood 2005;105(11):4527–31.

12. De Domenico I, Ward DM, Musci G, et al. Iron overload due to mutations in ferroportin. Haematologica 2006;91(1):92–5.

13. Drakesmith H, Schimanski LM, Ormerod E, et al. Resistance to hepcidin is conferred by hemochromatosis-associated mutations of ferroportin. Blood 2005;106(3):1092–7.

14. Allen KJ, Gurrin LC, Constantine CC, et al. Iron-overload-related disease in HFE hereditary hemochromatosis. N Engl J Med 2008;358(3):221–30.

15. Beutler E, Felitti VJ, Koziol JA, et al. Penetrance of 845G–> A (C282Y) HFE hereditary haemochromatosis mutation in the USA. Lancet 2002;359(9302):211–8.

16. EASL. EASL clinical practice guidelines for HFE hemochromatosis. J Hepatol 2010;53(1):3–22.

17. Moirand R, Adams PC, Bicheler V, et al. Clinical features of genetic hemochromatosis in women compared with men. Ann Intern Med 1997;127(2):105–10.

18. Loreal O, Deugnier Y, Moirand R, et al. Liver fibrosis in genetic hemochromatosis. Respective roles of iron and non-iron-related factors in 127 homozygous patients. J Hepatol 1992;16(1–2):122–7.

19. Desgrippes R, Laine F, Morcet J, et al. Decreased iron burden in overweight C282Y homozygous women: putative role of increased hepcidin production. Hepatology 2013;57(5):1784–92.

20. Milet J, Dehais V, Bourgain C, et al. Common variants in the BMP2, BMP4, and HJV genes of the hepcidin regulation pathway modulate HFE hemochromatosis penetrance. Am J Hum Genet 2007;81(4):799–807.

21. Stickel F, Buch S, Zoller H, et al. Evaluation of genome-wide loci of iron metabolism in hereditary hemochromatosis identifies PCSK7 as a host risk factor of liver cirrhosis. Hum Mol Genet 2014. [Epub ahead of print].

22. Adams PC, Reboussin DM, Press RD, et al. Biological variability of transferrin saturation and unsaturated iron-binding capacity. Am J Med 2007;120(11): 999.e1–7.

23. Niederau C, Fischer R, Purschel A, et al. Long-term survival in patients with hereditary hemochromatosis. Gastroenterology 1996;110(4):1107–19.

24. Beaton M, Guyader D, Deugnier Y, et al. Noninvasive prediction of cirrhosis in C282Y-linked hemochromatosis. Hepatology 2002;36(3):673–8.
25. Crawford DH, Murphy TL, Ramm LE, et al. Serum hyaluronic acid with serum ferritin accurately predicts cirrhosis and reduces the need for liver biopsy in C282Y hemochromatosis. Hepatology 2009;49(2):418–25.
26. Guyader D, Jacquelinet C, Moirand R, et al. Noninvasive prediction of fibrosis in C282Y homozygous hemochromatosis. Gastroenterology 1998;115(4):929–36.
27. Murphy CJ, Oudit GY. Iron-overload cardiomyopathy: pathophysiology, diagnosis, and treatment. J Card Fail 2010;16(11):888–900.
28. Le Lan C, Mosser A, Ropert M, et al. Sex and acquired cofactors determine phenotypes of ferroportin disease. Gastroenterology 2011;140(4):1199–207.e1–2.
29. Feder JN, Gnirke A, Thomas W, et al. A novel MHC class I-like gene is mutated in patients with hereditary haemochromatosis. Nat Genet 1996;13(4):399–408.
30. Walsh A, Dixon JL, Ramm GA, et al. The clinical relevance of compound heterozygosity for the C282Y and H63D substitutions in hemochromatosis. Clin Gastroenterol Hepatol 2006;4(11):1403–10.
31. Aguilar-Martinez P, Grandchamp B, Cunat S, et al. Iron overload in HFE C282Y heterozygotes at first genetic testing: a strategy for identifying rare HFE variants. Haematologica 2011;96(4):507–14.
32. Papanikolaou G, Samuels ME, Ludwig EH, et al. Mutations in HFE2 cause iron overload in chromosome 1q-linked juvenile hemochromatosis. Nat Genet 2004; 36(1):77–82.
33. Roetto A, Papanikolaou G, Politou M, et al. Mutant antimicrobial peptide hepcidin is associated with severe juvenile hemochromatosis. Nat Genet 2003;33(1):21–2.
34. Piperno A, Roetto A, Mariani R, et al. Homozygosity for transferrin receptor-2 Y250X mutation induces early iron overload. Haematologica 2004;89(3):359–60.
35. Bardou-Jacquet E, Cunat S, Beaumont-Epinette MP, et al. Variable age of onset and clinical severity in transferrin receptor 2 related haemochromatosis: novel observations. Br J Haematol 2013;162(2):278–81.
36. Njajou OT, Vaessen N, Joosse M, et al. A mutation in SLC11A3 is associated with autosomal dominant hemochromatosis. Nat Genet 2001;28(3):213–4.
37. Detivaud L, Island ML, Jouanolle AM, et al. Ferroportin diseases: functional studies, a link between genetic and clinical phenotype. Hum Mutat 2013; 34(11):1529–36.
38. Drakesmith H, Prentice AM. Hepcidin and the iron-infection axis. Science 2012; 338(6108):768–72.
39. Miyajima H, Takahashi Y, Kono S. Aceruloplasminemia, an inherited disorder of iron metabolism. Biometals 2003;16(1):205–13.
40. Kautz L, Jung G, Nemeth E, et al. The erythroid factor erythroferrone and its role in iron homeostasis [abstract]. Blood 2013;122(21):4.

Iron-Refractory Iron Deficiency Anemia (IRIDA)

Matthew M. Heeney, MD[a], Karin E. Finberg, MD, PhD[b],*

KEYWORDS

- Iron-refractory iron deficiency anemia • Inherited iron deficiency • Hepcidin
- *TMPRSS6* • Matriptase-2

KEY POINTS

- Iron-refractory iron deficiency anemia (IRIDA) is an inherited disorder of systemic iron balance in which both absorption and utilization of iron are impaired.
- Patients with IRIDA show iron deficiency anemia that is refractory to oral iron therapy but partially responsive to parenteral iron.
- IRIDA is caused by mutations in the gene *TMPRSS6*.
- *TMPRSS6* encodes matriptase-2, a transmembrane serine protease expressed by the liver that regulates the production of the iron regulatory hormone hepcidin.
- Studies conducted in tissue culture systems and mouse models have enhanced our understanding of the underlying pathogenesis.

INTRODUCTION

Iron is an essential metal for many biologic processes in mammals. Its primary role is to bind oxygen in the heme moiety of hemoglobin. Iron also plays a central role in the enzymatic transfer of electrons performed by cytochromes, peroxidases, ribonucleotide reductases, and catalases. This reactivity of iron also has the potential to cause damage to biologic systems if iron is "free" and not bound and transported by a finely regulated and complex system of proteins that maintain iron homeostasis.

Under normal physiologic conditions in the adult male, only 1 to 2 mg of the 20 to 25 mg of iron required daily to maintain erythropoiesis enters the body through carefully regulated intestinal absorption.[1] Most of the daily iron need is derived from the recycling of erythroid iron through phagocytosis of senescent red cells by

Funding Sources: None (M.M. Heeney); National Institutes of Health K08 DK084204, Burroughs Wellcome Fund Career Award for Medical Scientists (K.E. Finberg).
Conflict of Interest: None.
a Dana-Farber/Boston Children's Cancer and Blood Disorders Center, 300 Longwood Avenue, Boston, MA 02115, USA; b Department of Pathology, Yale School of Medicine, 310 Cedar Street, New Haven, CT 06510, USA
* Corresponding author.
E-mail address: karin.finberg@yale.edu

Hematol Oncol Clin N Am 28 (2014) 637–652
http://dx.doi.org/10.1016/j.hoc.2014.04.009
0889-8588/14/$ – see front matter © 2014 Elsevier Inc. All rights reserved.

reticuloendothelial macrophages and degradation of hemoglobin. As humans have no physiologically regulated mechanism for excreting iron from the body, control of iron balance occurs almost entirely at the level of intestinal absorption.

Virtually all plasma iron exists bound to the circulating glycoprotein transferrin (TF), which allows the iron to remain soluble, renders iron nonreactive, and facilitates its cellular import through the transferrin cycle.[2] Iron-loaded plasma transferrin binds to transferrin receptors (TFR) on the cell surface. The TF/TFR receptor complex is endocytosed, and acidification of the endosome results in the release of iron from TF. The iron is transported out of the endosome into the cytoplasm, and the empty TF and TFR return to the cell surface and are released into the plasma to repeat this cycle.

Most nonerythroid intracellular iron is stored in hepatocytes and macrophages in the form of ferritin, a multimeric iron storage protein whose structure facilitates iron bioavailability in response to cellular need. Intracellular iron, either absorbed by the duodenal enterocyte or liberated by macrophages from heme recycling, is either stored as ferritin or exported into the plasma by ferroportin.[3] Ferroportin, which is the sole known mammalian cellular iron exporter, is highly expressed on the basolateral membrane of enterocytes and on the cell membrane of reticuloendothelial macrophages.

Iron homeostasis requires carefully coordinated regulation of intestinal iron absorption, cellular iron import/export, and iron storage. Hepcidin, a small circulating peptide released by the liver, is the master regulator of systemic iron balance. Hepcidin limits both iron absorption from the intestine and iron release from macrophage stores by binding to ferroportin and triggering ferroportin's internalization and degradation. Hepcidin expression is modulated in response to several physiologic and pathophysiological stimuli, which include systemic iron loading, erythropoietic activity, and inflammation.[4]

As is the case with many physiologic processes, spontaneous mutations leading to disease in animals and humans have revealed much about the normal regulation of iron transport and storage in humans. In particular, the identification of TMPRSS6 as the gene mutated in cases of iron-refractory iron deficiency anemia (IRIDA), has increased our knowledge of the molecular mechanisms that regulate hepcidin expression.

CLINICAL PRESENTATION

In 1981, Buchanan and Sheehan[5] described 3 siblings with iron deficiency anemia despite adequate dietary iron intake and no evidence of gastrointestinal blood loss. All 3 failed to respond to oral ferrous sulfate therapy. In 2 of the siblings, a formal oral iron "challenge" (see **Box 2**) to assess for impaired intestinal iron absorption failed to show evidence of a rise in serum iron 2 hours after the oral administration of 2 mg/kg elemental iron as ferrous sulfate. Following intramuscular injection of iron dextran, the 3 siblings also showed only a partial hematological response assessed by hemoglobin and red cell indices. In addition, although intramuscular iron administration raised the serum ferritin level, suggesting restoration of iron stores, the patients nevertheless remained hypoferremic. The investigators postulated that the phenotype was explained in part by an inherited, iron-specific absorptive defect, which was further compounded by a defect of iron utilization reflected in the partial response to parenteral iron therapy.

Pearson and Lukens[6] subsequently described 2 affected siblings. In addition to recognizing the intestinal iron uptake defect reflected in the failed response to oral iron challenge, these investigators also documented a discordance in the rate of decline of transferrin saturation (rapid) and serum ferritin (slower) after iron dextran administration. Given that iron dextran must be phagocytosed and "recycled" by macrophages before the iron can be made available for erythropoiesis, the investigators postulated that a macrophage iron retention phenotype/macrophage iron recycling defect contributed to the phenotype.

Further cases of familial iron deficiency anemia with similar clinical presentations were subsequently reported, which provided additional insight into the mode of genetic transmission as well as the underlying pathophysiological defect.[7–11] Brown and colleagues[8] reported 2 affected female siblings of Northern European ancestry whose parents exhibited normal hematological parameters, thus suggesting a recessive mode of transmission for the disorder. Galanello and colleagues[11] provided additional evidence for autosomal recessive transmission in a large kindred that originated in a small village in southern Sardinia; the structure of this pedigree, which contained 5 affected individuals, suggested that the disorder might be caused by homozygosity for a mutation that arose in a common ancestor. Hartman and Barker[9] reported an affected African American sibling pair in whom bone marrow biopsies performed after parenteral iron therapy failed to demonstrate normal sideroblasts (erythroid normoblasts containing stainable nonhemoglobin iron in the cytoplasm), despite the presence of stainable iron in bone marrow macrophages. This observation thus provided evidence in support of the iron utilization defect that had been postulated by Buchanan and Sheehan.[5]

Review of these case reports identified several unifying features that suggested that these cases represented the same underlying disorder, a condition that has been termed iron-refractory iron deficiency anemia (IRIDA).[12] These key features of IRIDA include (**Box 1**) (1) congenital hypochromic, microcytic anemia (hemoglobin 6–9 g/dL); (2) very low mean corpuscular volume (45–65 fL); (3) very low transferrin saturation (<5%); (4) abnormal oral iron absorption (as indicated by a lack of hematological improvement following treatment with oral iron or failure of an oral iron challenge); (5) abnormal iron utilization (as indicated by a sluggish, incomplete, and transient response to parenteral iron); and (6) an inheritance pattern compatible with autosomal recessive transmission. In these cases, acquired causes of iron deficiency (eg, gastrointestinal blood loss) and inherited causes of microcytosis (eg, thalassemias, lead toxicity) were excluded by extensive laboratory testing. Furthermore, no case showed clinical evidence of a chronic inflammatory disorder or generalized

---

Box 1
Key clinical features and typical laboratory data from untreated IRIDA probands at diagnosis in childhood

- Lifelong/congenital, usually presents in childhood
- Severe microcytosis (mean corpuscular volume 45–65 fL)
- Moderate/severe anemia (hemoglobin 6–9 g/dL)
- Severe hypoferremia with very low transferrin saturation (<5%)
- No or minimal response to oral iron supplementation
- Abnormal oral iron absorption/failure of an oral iron challenge
- Incomplete and transient response to parenteral iron
- Autosomal recessive transmission
- Anemia often ameliorates into adulthood, although hypoferremia persists

intestinal malabsorptive defect. Hemoglobinopathies and sideroblastic anemias were excluded as potential causes of the microcytosis by hemoglobin electrophoresis and bone marrow examinations, respectively.

In the published IRIDA cases, subjects were generally healthy and growing normally, and the anemia was typically detected during routine screening usually conducted before the age of 2 years. Thus, from the clinical histories, it was not known if patients with IRIDA were already iron-deficient at birth. Of note, the proband reported by Brown and colleagues,[8] who was diagnosed with microcytic anemia at age 9 months, showed plentiful reticuloendothelial iron stores on an initial bone marrow examination performed after a 3-month failed course of oral iron therapy but showed an absence of stainable iron on repeat bone marrow examination performed at age 4 years after a course of intramuscular iron. These findings, along with reports of normal birth weights for IRIDA patients,[10] raise the possibility that in utero iron transfer may be normal in these patients, with the depletion of iron stores occurring only after birth.[13]

For unclear reasons, the clinical signs and symptoms of IRIDA appear distinct from severe acquired iron deficiency anemia. Although IRIDA subjects have laboratory evidence of severe iron deficiency, clinical signs observed in acquired iron deficiency have been noted inconsistently in the reported IRIDA cases. Moderate to severe pallor was described in the kindred reported by Melis and colleagues.[14] The 18-month-old proband reported by Andrews[10] was described as pale with dry skin. Studying the kindred originally reported by Brown and colleagues,[8] Pearson and Lukens[6] noted that the affected siblings developed angular cheilitis (crusted, painful lesions at corners of their mouths) that receded after intravenous iron therapy. Only rarely are signs and symptoms associated with iron deficiency, such as koilonychias or hair loss, described in IRIDA.[15] Although IRIDA has been considered a rare clinical entity based on the small number of cases reported in the literature, it is possible that in the absence of routine laboratory screening for anemia, many cases never come to clinical attention because of the normal growth and development of the affected individuals. Remarkably, despite congenital, severe iron deficiency, long-term follow-up of the affected subjects has shown normal growth and normal intellectual development,[6,14] with no evidence of the cognitive concerns on which iron deficiency screening in infancy have been founded.[16]

Given the small number of reported cases, experience with the natural history and long-term management of IRIDA is, at present, limited. Pearson and Lukens[6] proposed a treatment regimen that involved the parenteral administration of iron dextran every 2 to 4 years, or when serum ferritin levels fell below 50 to 75 ng/mL or the mouth ulcerations observed in their patients recurred. Hartman and colleagues[17] described the course of 5 patients with IRIDA who had been followed for 15 years. They noted that repeated iron infusions that elevated the serum ferritin to levels greater than 200 ng/mL resulted in considerable improvement in both the anemia and microcytosis. Although the serum iron and transferrin saturation occasionally reached the normal range, the patients generally developed recurrent hypoferremia. With the cessation of iron infusions, microcytosis returned, but not to the severe degree present in infancy. In the affected family members studied by Galanello and colleagues (who on last report range from 18 to 48 years of age), the anemia was more severe during childhood, requiring intermittent intravenous iron administration. However, hemoglobin levels of 10.0 to 13.9 g/dL were maintained in the adult affected subjects, although laboratory findings of iron-restricted erythropoiesis (low mean corpuscular volume, low mean corpuscular hemoglobin, low serum iron, low transferrin saturation) persisted. In addition to a relative amelioration of anemia into adulthood, serum ferritin levels also appeared to rise with age in this kindred. The investigators suggested that the increased severity of the anemia during childhood could indicate the greater iron demands for body growth and for the accompanying expansion of the red cell mass that occurs during this period; in adulthood, however, a larger proportion of the limited iron available could be used in erythropoiesis.[14]

GENETICS

Strong evidence that the IRIDA phenotype has an inherited basis was obtained through genetic characterization of a large, consanguineous kindred from Sardinia. In this kindred, in which disease in affected individuals could be attributed to homozygosity for a mutation arising in a common ancestor, the IRIDA phenotype mapped to the long arm of chromosome 22 (22q12.3–13.1) under a model of recessive inheritance.[18] IRIDA subsequently was shown to be caused by mutations in the gene *TMPRSS6*,[12,14] which resides within this critical region of chromosome 22q and for which a key role in iron balance had recently been revealed through study of the orthologous gene in mice (see later in this article).[19] Notably, patients with the IRIDA phenotype showed levels of hepcidin in their serum, plasma, and/or urine that were indicative of impaired hepcidin regulation.[12,14,20] Although hepcidin levels are normally reduced in response to systemic iron deficiency (an adaptive response to promote absorption of dietary iron),[21,22] patients with IRIDA displayed hepcidin levels that were either within or above the reference range. Given the known ability of hepcidin to limit ferroportin-dependent iron export from enterocytes and macrophages,[4] the inappropriately elevated hepcidin levels in IRIDA provide insight into the iron refractory features of the disorder. Specifically, the inappropriate hepcidin excess in IRIDA can explain (1) the development of systemic iron deficiency as a result of impaired absorption of dietary iron, (2) the failure to achieve a hematological response to oral iron therapies, and (3) the sluggish and incomplete utilization of parental iron formulations, which consist of iron-carbohydrate complexes that require processing by macrophages before the iron can be used in erythropoiesis. In many respects, IRIDA can be considered the pathophysiologic and phenotypic opposite of hereditary hemochromatosis, in which the "uncoupling" of appropriate hepcidin expression from the sensing of iron stores results in an inappropriate hepcidin "deficiency" (see the article by Brissot, elsewhere in this issue).

TMPRSS6 (transmembrane protease, serine 6) encodes matriptase-2, a membrane-spanning protease that is primarily expressed by the liver.[23] Matriptase-2 is a member of the type II transmembrane serine protease (TTSP) family, a group that is anchored to the membrane at their amino termini. The protein name, matriptase-2, reflects structural homology to another TTSP, matriptase-1. Matriptase-2 contains a large extracellular region containing several structural domains, including an SEA (sea urchin sperm protein, enteropeptidase, agrin) domain, 2 CUB (C1r/C1s, urchin embryonic growth factor, bone morphogenetic protein 1) domains, 3 LDLRA (low-density lipoprotein receptor class A) domains, and a C-terminal catalytic domain containing a classic catalytic triad of serine, histidine, and aspartic acid residues (**Fig. 1**). Matriptase-2 is believed to be synthesized as an inactive, membrane-bound, single-chain polypeptide that undergoes a complex series of proteolytic cleavage events during zymogen activation.[24] When overexpressed in cultured cells, matriptase-2 localizes to the plasma membrane[23] and is shed from the cell surface as an activated, 2-chain form.[25] Recombinant matriptase-2 has been shown in vitro to degrade components of the extracellular matrix and basement membrane, such as fibrinogen, fibronectin, and type I collagen.[23] Interestingly, overexpression of matriptase-2 in breast and prostate cancer cell lines can reduce their

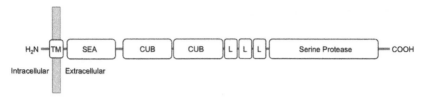

Fig. 1. Schematic representation of the domain structure of matriptase-2. Labeled are the transmembrane (TM), complement factor C1r/C1s, urchin embryonic growth factor, and bone morphogenetic protein (CUB), LDL-receptor class A (L), and serine protease domains.

invasive properties in vitro, suggesting a possible role for matriptase-2 in cancer development and progression.[26]

A key role for *TMPRSS6* in iron homeostasis was first revealed through elucidation of the genetic basis of a chemically induced, recessive mutant mouse phenotype termed *mask*.[19] The *mask* mutant received its name because it showed progressive loss of truncal hair but retained hair on the head. Notably, mice with the *mask* phenotype also exhibited microcytic anemia, low plasma iron levels, and low iron stores when raised on a standard rodent laboratory diet. Furthermore, *mask* mice showed evidence of defective hepcidin regulation in the setting of iron deficiency. Although control mice suppressed hepatic hepcidin production in response to a low-iron diet (an appropriate physiologic response to promote iron absorption), hepcidin messenger RNA (mRNA) levels in livers of *mask* mutants were inappropriately elevated. Genetic mapping of the underlying mutation revealed that *mask* mice were homozygous for a mutation that resulted in defective splicing of the *Tmprss6* transcript, which eliminated the proteolytic domain of matriptase-2. The elevated hepcidin mRNA levels detected in the livers of the *mask* mutants suggest that the normal function of the *Tmprss6* gene product, matriptase-2, is to lower hepcidin expression by the liver.

A *Tmprss6* knockout (*Tmprss6$^{-/-}$*) mouse, generated by standard gene-targeting techniques, exhibited a phenotype very similar to the *mask Tmprss6* splicing mutant, including the key feature of hepatic hepcidin overexpression.[27] Notably, the anemia and alopecia phenotypes of both the engineered and the chemically induced *Tmprss6* mutants could be rescued by iron administration.[19,27] Consistent with the known ability of hepcidin to promote ferroportin internalization and degradation, duodenal enterocytes of *Tmprss6$^{-/-}$* mice showed decreased ferroportin protein expression in the basolateral membrane that was accompanied by histologic evidence of iron retention within these cells.[27] Thus, in the setting of hepcidin elevation, when basolateral export of iron into the plasma is restricted, iron accumulates within duodenal enterocytes and is ultimately lost from the body when these cells are shed into the gut lumen.

Studies conducted in tissue culture systems and transgenic models have begun to shed insight into the mechanism by which matriptase-2 regulates hepcidin production. This mechanism appears to involve modulation of bone morphogenetic protein (BMP)/SMAD signaling, a key signal transduction pathway that promotes hepcidin transcription in hepatocytes (**Fig. 2**). BMPs are secreted ligands of the transforming growth factor β superfamily that interact with type 1 and type 2 BMP receptors at the cell membrane to trigger the phosphorylation of multiple receptor-associated SMAD proteins (SMAD1, SMAD5, SMAD8). Once phosphorylated, these receptor-associated SMADs bind to a common mediator, SMAD4, forming heterodimeric complexes that translocate to the nucleus to regulate transcription of BMP target genes, including the gene encoding hepcidin, by binding to specific elements in the promoters of genes.[28] Of note, signaling through the BMP pathway is modulated in

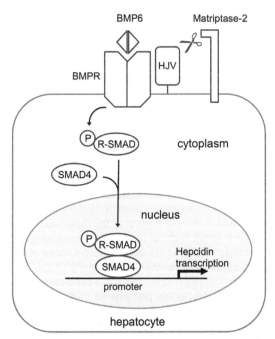

Fig. 2. Model of hepcidin regulation by matriptase-2. The binding of BMP ligands to BMP receptor complexes (BMPRs) at the hepatocyte plasma membrane initiates an intracellular signaling cascade that promotes hepcidin transcription. BMP6 appears to be the particular BMP family ligand that plays a key role in initiating this signaling in vivo. BMP6 binding to BMPRs induces phosphorylation (P) of receptor-associated SMAD proteins (R-SMADs). Once phosphorylated, R-SMADs form a complex with the common mediator SMAD4. This SMAD complex then translocates to the nucleus to bind specific target elements in the promoter of the hepcidin gene to increase hepcidin expression. The *TMPRSS6* gene product, matriptase-2, dampens signal transduction through this pathway by cleaving hemojuvelin (HJV), a BMP co-receptor, from the plasma membrane.

response to hepatic iron stores. When local iron stores increase, the liver raises expression of BMP6, the particular BMP ligand that appears to play a key role in promoting hepcidin transcription. This leads to increased hepcidin expression, an adaptive response to limit further iron absorption from the diet.[29–31]

Matriptase-2 has been shown to inhibit BMP signaling, and thus hepcidin transcription, by cleaving a glycosylphosphatidylinositol-linked protein termed hemojuvelin from the cell membrane.[32] Hemojuvelin, which functions as a co-receptor for BMP ligands,[33] plays a key role in promoting hepatic BMP signaling, as evidenced by the fact that loss-of-function mutations in the hemojuvelin gene result in juvenile hemochromatosis, a severe form of hereditary iron overload that is associated with inappropriately low levels of hepcidin.[34] In cultured cells, the ability of recombinant matriptase-2 to cleave hemojuvelin has been shown to be impaired by missense mutation of the matriptase-2 catalytic domain and to be abolished by a matriptase-2 truncating mutation that eliminates the catalytic domain entirely.[32] Additionally, mice with genetic disruption of *Tmprss6* show low hepatic iron stores accompanied by up-regulated hepatic expression of Bmp target genes, phenotypic features that are dependent on the presence of both the Bmp6 ligand and the Bmp co-receptor hemojuvelin.[35–37] Collectively, these findings suggest that the hepcidin elevation observed in patents with the

IRIDA phenotype results from an inability to appropriately down-regulate hepatic BMP signaling in the context of low hepatic iron stores.

Given that the presence of functional matriptase-2 appears to prevent hepcidin overexpression, it has been proposed that changes in matriptase-2 protein levels or protein activity may serve as a means to regulate hepcidin production. Indeed, in studies conducted in cultured cells and/or animal models, a variety of stimuli with known capacity to modulate hepcidin expression have been found capable of modulating *TMPRSS6* mRNA and/or matriptase-2 protein levels. The stimuli include hypoxia,[38,39] acute dietary iron restriction,[40] chronic dietary iron loading,[41] BMP6 injection,[41] and inflammation.[42] Future studies may elucidate how these various stimuli interact to collectively orchestrate matriptase-2 expression.

To date, at least 45 different *TMPRSS6* mutations have reported in individuals with the IRIDA phenotype. These include 20 missense mutations, 5 nonsense mutations, 10 frameshift mutations, 1 large in-frame deletion, and 9 intronic mutations predicted to disrupt normal splicing.[12,14,15,20,43–56] Most of the reported mutations are unique to single families, whereas a small number have been found to recur in 2 or more kindreds. Mutations have been identified in kindreds from a range of ethnic backgrounds, without evidence for a significant founder effect. Many of the *TMPRSS6* mutations detected in patients with the IRIDA phenotype are predicted to impair matriptase-2 proteolytic activity. For example, some pathogenic mutations generate truncated or aberrantly spliced *TMPRSS6* transcripts, whereas others introduce missense substitutions in the catalytic domain. *TMPRSS6* missense mutations are not restricted to the proteolytic domain, however, and functional analyses have revealed how missense substitutions in other matriptase-2 domains can also ultimately result in impaired hemojuvelin cleavage activity. For example, missense mutations in the second LDLRA domain have been shown to impair matriptase-2 trafficking to the plasma membrane,[43] whereas a missense mutation in the SEA domain has been shown to impair activation of the protease.[15]

TMPRSS6 mutations are routinely sought by polymerase chain reaction–based DNA sequencing, an approach that typically examines all coding regions (ie, exons and intron/exon boundaries) of a gene. To date, most individuals who exhibit the IRIDA phenotype have been found to possess either 2 different *TMPRSS6* mutations in compound heterozygosity (ie, inherited from different parents) or a single mutation in homozygous form. However, affected individuals from several unrelated kindreds also have been reported who have each been found to harbor only a single, heterozygous *TMPRSS6* mutation.[12,53] It is possible that such individuals may harbor a second mutation on the other *TMPRSS6* allele in an unanalyzed noncoding region that is important for *TMPRSS6* gene regulation (such as an intronic or promoter region), but this has yet to be demonstrated. In some reported kindreds, microcytic anemia has been observed in the parent of a child exhibiting the classic IRIDA phenotype, raising the possibility that heterozygosity for *TMPRSS6* mutation may increase the susceptibility to iron deficiency anemia in some settings.[52] Indeed, in mice that are heterozygous for *Tmprss6* mutation, systemic iron homeostasis is mildly compromised.[36,57]

To date, *TMPRSS6* is the only gene in which mutations are known to result in the IRIDA phenotype. Although *TMPRSS6* genotype-phenotype correlations in IRIDA have not yet been extensively studied, some investigators have noted a tendency toward lower hemoglobin, lower erythrocyte mean corpuscular volume, and lower serum transferrin saturation in affected individuals harboring 2 nonsense mutations compared with those harboring either 2 missense mutations or 1 missense and 1 nonsense mutation.[13] Notably, although the IRIDA phenotype associated with *TMPRSS6* mutations was originally defined to include the inability to respond to oral iron therapy,[12] several individuals with biallelic *TMPRSS6* mutations who have been reported subsequently have shown a partial correction of anemia with prolonged or sustained administration of oral iron.[43,51,54,55] In one of these kindreds, the affected siblings presented with microcytic anemia, hypoferremia, and, interestingly, hyperferritinemia before the initiation of oral iron therapy.[54] Thus, it is becoming evident that the phenotypic spectrum of disease associated with *TMPRSS6* mutations extends beyond the classic IRIDA phenotype, and this spectrum of presentations should be recognized during the clinical evaluation of iron deficiency anemia.

In addition to the rare pathogenic *TMPRSS6* mutations that have been associated with IRIDA, several common variants (ie, single nucleotide polymorphisms [SNPs]) in *TMPRSS6* have also been described in multiple global populations.[58,59] Genome-wide association studies conducted in several large populations have correlated these SNPs at the *TMPRSS6* locus with several laboratory parameters related to iron status, such as hemoglobin level, mean corpuscular volume, mean corpuscular hemoglobin, serum iron level, and serum transferrin saturation.[60–65] One of the *TMPRSS6* SNPs showing the strongest associations to these parameters, rs855791, encodes an alanine-to-valine substitution at position 736 within the matriptase-2 serine protease domain (p.Ala736Val). Compared with the alanine-containing variant, matriptase-2 possessing a valine at position 736 was found to be less effective in suppressing hepcidin levels in vitro, and p.Ala736Val was also shown to associate with serum hepcidin levels in a large Italian population from which subjects with iron deficiency and inflammation had been excluded.[66] Although these findings suggest that the association of *TMPRSS6* polymorphisms with laboratory parameters of iron status may result from an intermediate effect of these polymorphisms on hepcidin expression, 2 population-based studies interestingly have found that the associations of *TMPRSS6* SNPs with iron and erythrocyte parameters are at least partly independent of hepcidin levels.[67,68]

The key role of matriptase-2 in dampening hepcidin production through the BMP/SMAD pathway has raised the possibility that inhibition of *TMPRSS6* activity could be used as a therapeutic strategy to increase hepcidin expression, and therefore reduce iron loading, in certain clinical disorders in which iron loading results from hepcidin insufficiency. In proof-of-principle studies, genetic disruption of *Tmprss6* has been shown to reduce iron loading in mouse models of *HFE*-associated hereditary hemochromatosis[69] and β-thalassemia intermedia.[70] In humans, milder changes in matriptase-2 activity resulting from *TMPRSS6* polymorphisms have been suggested to influence the phenotypic expression of several clinical disorders associated with abnormalities of iron homeostasis. For example, the *TMPRSS6* p.Ala736Val variant has been found to correlate with serum transferrin saturation and serum ferritin levels in patients with hereditary hemochromatosis,[71] with serum hepcidin levels and erythropoietin requirements in patients undergoing chronic hemodialysis,[72] and with hepatic iron accumulation in patients with nonalcoholic fatty liver disease.[73]

DIFFERENTIAL DIAGNOSIS

The differential diagnosis of microcytic hypochromic anemia is dominated by acquired iron deficiency resulting from either poor dietary intake or ongoing losses. Similarly, for congenital microcytic hypochromic anemias, the differential diagnosis is dominated by the thalassemia syndromes. The approach to the diagnosis of rarer forms of congenital microcytic anemias has been recently reviewed.[74] In addition to the congenital defect in iron absorption that underlies IRIDA, these rarer congenital microcytic anemias result from defects in iron transport, iron uptake, and mitochondrial iron utilization (see the article about sideroblastic anemia by Bottomley, elsewhere in this issue).

The prevalence of the rare congenital microcytic anemias is not easily determined. However, the recent increase in published IRIDA cases and affected families suggests that IRIDA may be the most common form. An approach to the diagnosis of IRIDA is shown in **Fig. 3**. Once iron deficiency is confirmed, the algorithm must start with a rigorous exclusion of the acquired causes of iron deficiency (eg, blood loss, iron-poor diet, and long-standing inflammatory conditions). Clues for an IRIDA diagnosis

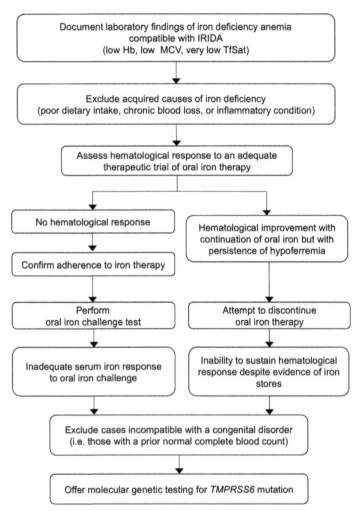

Fig. 3. Diagnostic algorithm for the clinical evaluation of IRIDA. Suspicion for IRIDA should arise in a subject with a lifelong significant microcytic hypochromic anemia and biochemical evidence of iron deficiency without a history of inadequate iron intake or ongoing iron/blood loss. If the iron deficiency anemia does not respond to oral iron supplementation and/or has an incomplete/transient response to parenteral iron therapy, an oral iron challenge will assess for impaired intestinal iron absorption from either intestinal pathology or an inappropriately high hepcidin state. Hb, hemoglobin; IDA, iron deficiency anemia; IRIDA, Iron-Refractory Iron Deficiency Anemia; MCV, mean corpuscular volume; TfSat, transferrin saturation.

from the initial assessment of iron status in an untreated subject include 2 patterns: (1) the degree of microcytosis (mean corpuscular volume [MCV] 45–65 fL range) relative to the anemia (hemoglobin [Hb] 6–8 g/dL range); and (2) a profound hypoferremia and low transferrin saturation (usually <5%) relative to a slightly low or even normal ferritin. Most commonly, subjects with iron deficiency will be treated with an empiric course of adequate iron supplementation. Poor or absent response to oral iron supplementation is most commonly associated with poor adherence to therapy, inadequate dosing, or inadequate duration of therapy. If these common pitfalls can be avoided and an adequate oral trial fails to produce a hematologic benefit, one must consider the possibility of impaired intestinal iron absorption.

Efficient intestinal iron absorption requires an acidic duodenal environment and a functioning duodenal epithelium. Common reasons for poor iron absorption include achlorhydria due to chronic proton pump inhibition and damage to the duodenum (eg, celiac sprue). States of elevated hepcidin, which include anemia of chronic inflammation, as well as IRIDA, result in impaired export of iron from the duodenal enterocyte into the plasma. In the hypoferremic patient, an oral iron challenge (**Box 2**) can identify inadequate iron absorption; however, the test does not distinguish the etiology and may prompt more aggressive gastrointestinal evaluation.

If the oral iron challenge suggests inadequate absorption and the iron deficiency truly appears to have onset in infancy or childhood, IRIDA is a more likely diagnosis. The only current diagnostic test for IRIDA is sequencing of the *TMPRSS6* gene. Ideally, clinicians could determine the plasma or urinary hepcidin and easily distinguish true iron deficiency (based on a finding of low hepcidin) from IRIDA (in which hepcidin would be inappropriately high). However, although more than a decade has passed since the discovery of hepcidin, there is yet no hepcidin assay approved by the Food and Drug Administration available for clinical use. Once a hepcidin assay becomes available, it may serve as a useful aid in the diagnosis of IRIDA.

Box 2
Oral iron challenge

In the hypoferremic patient, this simple and minimally invasive test distinguishes an intestinal iron absorption defect from other causes of chronic iron deficiency. There are no systematically validated, published procedures or expected response criteria for an oral iron challenge test. The procedure that follows is largely based on our clinical experience and data published in individual case reports.[77,78]

Procedure:

A. Ideally the subject should be fasting for at least 6 hours.

B. Draw blood samples for serum iron, transferrin (TIBC), and ferritin.

C. Ferrous sulfate (eg, Fer-in-Sol) 4–6 mg/kg of elemental iron PO.

D. Redraw blood samples for serum iron at 90 minutes post dose (some perform repeated sampling every 30 minutes for up to 3 hours post oral dose).

Interpretation:

In a hypoferremic subject capable of absorbing iron from the intestine, the serum iron level is expected to increase by at least 50 μg/dL 90 minutes after the oral iron challenge. Failure of a fasting subject to achieve an appropriate increase in serum iron level is indicative of a defect in intestinal iron absorption. For nonfasting subjects, an equivocal rise in serum iron would not be readily interpretable; however, the test results would remain interpretable if either a substantial increase in the serum iron level or no change in the serum iron level whatsoever were observed.

TREATMENT

The mainstay of therapy for IRIDA is intermittent parenteral iron supplementation. In many case reports and series, parenteral iron has been demonstrated to improve the anemia in the IRIDA phenotype. However, the hemoglobin response to parenteral iron is usually not completely corrective and is of shorter duration than expected in most cases. Depending on the formulation and dose limitations, repeated dosing is usually required and can become onerous. Although many parenteral iron formulations have been used with efficacy, the optimal formulation and frequency of dosing has not been determined. Although not yet described, the concern with repeated parenteral iron dosing would be for iron overload; however, given the inappropriately high hepcidin levels in IRIDA, one would expect a hemosiderosis pattern of reticuloendothelial macrophage loading rather than parenchymal loading.

Given that the classic IRIDA phenotype includes absent/minimal response to an oral iron challenge, there does not seem to be a significant role for oral iron supplementation in IRIDA. However, Cau and colleagues[75] recently described a child with homozygous *TMPRSS6* splice site mutation (IVS6+1 G>C) who demonstrated the classical unresponsiveness to oral iron therapy and partial response to parenteral therapy, yet had a remarkable response with the addition of ascorbic acid to the ferrous sulfate oral supplement. The investigators noted that the addition of ascorbic acid was not effective in the affected adults in the family, and they hypothesized that the increased iron needs of the rapidly growing child explained the differential benefit observed between age groups.

The addition of recombinant erythropoietin has been described by several groups but has not shown significant benefit in IRIDA.[15,56] The rationale for erythropoietin supplementation was that in high doses it can provide some benefit in the high hepcidin state of anemia of chronic inflammation. However, as shown by Lehmberg and colleagues,[56] administration of recombinant human erythropoietin up to 273 U/kg per week alone did not improve anemia.

In a recent case report, a hematologic response to glucocorticoid therapy was reported in a child with hypochromic microcytic anemia who had shown little response to oral therapy and who also had an elevated hepcidin level. However, given that sequencing of the *TMPRSS6* gene revealed only common polymorphisms (but not pathogenic *TMPRSS6* mutations) in this child, the relevance of this therapy for patients with IRIDA due to *TMPRSS6* mutations remains uncertain.[76]

Ultimately, optimally effective therapies may require manipulation of the inappropriately elevated hepcidin levels. There are currently several experimental agents in clinical trials for anemia of chronic inflammation that also could have benefit in treating the pathophysiology of IRIDA (see the article by Ganz, elsewhere in this issue).

ACKNOWLEDGMENTS

The authors acknowledge Drs Nancy C. Andrews and Mark D. Fleming for sparking their interests in the field of iron homeostasis and for providing continued outstanding mentorship.

REFERENCES

1. Cook JD, Barry WE, Hershko C, et al. Iron kinetics with emphasis on iron overload. Am J Pathol 1973;72(2):337–44.
2. Chen C, Paw BH. Cellular and mitochondrial iron homeostasis in vertebrates. Biochim Biophys Acta 2012;1823(9):1459–67.

3. Ward DM, Kaplan J. Ferroportin-mediated iron transport: expression and regulation. Biochim Biophys Acta 2012;1823(9):1426–33.
4. Ganz T. Systemic iron homeostasis. Physiol Rev 2013;93(4):1721–41.
5. Buchanan GR, Sheehan RG. Malabsorption and defective utilization of iron in three siblings. J Pediatr 1981;98(5):723–8.
6. Pearson HA, Lukens JN. Ferrokinetics in the syndrome of familial hypoferremic microcytic anemia with iron malabsorption. J Pediatr Hematol Oncol 1999;21:412–7.
7. Mayo MM, Samuel SM. Iron deficiency anemia due to a defect in iron metabolism: a case report. Clin Lab Sci 2001;14(3):135–8.
8. Brown AC, Lutton JD, Pearson HA, et al. Heme metabolism and in vitro erythropoiesis in anemia associated with hypochromic microcytosis. Am J Hematol 1988;27(1):1–6.
9. Hartman KR, Barker JA. Microcytic anemia with iron malabsorption: an inherited disorder of iron metabolism. Am J Hematol 1996;51(4):269–75.
10. Andrews NC. Iron deficiency: lessons from anemic mice. Yale J Biol Med 1997;70(3):219–26.
11. Galanello R, Cau M, Melis MA, et al. Studies of NRAMP2, transferrin receptor and transferrin genes as candidate genes for human hereditary microcytic anemia due to defective iron absorption and utilization [abstract]. Blood 1998;92(Suppl 1):669a.
12. Finberg KE, Heeney MM, Campagna DR, et al. Mutations in TMPRSS6 cause iron-refractory iron deficiency anemia (IRIDA). Nat Genet 2008;40(5):569–71.
13. De Falco L, Sanchez M, Silvestri L, et al. Iron refractory iron deficiency anemia. Haematologica 2013;98(6):845–53.
14. Melis MA, Cau M, Congiu R, et al. A mutation in the TMPRSS6 gene, encoding a transmembrane serine protease that suppresses hepcidin production, in familial iron deficiency anemia refractory to oral iron. Haematologica 2008;93(10):1473–9.
15. Ramsay AJ, Quesada V, Sanchez M, et al. Matriptase-2 mutations in iron-refractory iron deficiency anemia patients provide new insights into protease activation mechanisms. Hum Mol Genet 2009;18(19):3673–83.
16. Baker RD, Greer FR, Committee on Nutrition American Academy of Pediatrics. Diagnosis and prevention of iron deficiency and iron-deficiency anemia in infants and young children (0-3 years of age). Pediatrics 2010;126(5):1040–50.
17. Hartman KR, Finberg KE, Merino ME. Iron resistant iron deficiency anemia: long term follow-up of 5 patients [abstract]. ASPHO Annual Meeting Abstracts. San Diego, 2009.
18. Melis MA, Cau M, Congiu R, et al. Identification of a gene involved in hereditary microcytic anemia due to defective iron absorption in a Sardinian family [abstract]. Eur J Hum Genet 2007;15(S1):261.
19. Du X, She E, Gelbart T, et al. The serine protease TMPRSS6 is required to sense iron deficiency. Science 2008;320(5879):1088–92.
20. Guillem F, Lawson S, Kannengiesser C, et al. Two nonsense mutations in the TMPRSS6 gene in a patient with microcytic anemia and iron deficiency. Blood 2008;112(5):2089–91.
21. Kemna EH, Tjalsma H, Podust VN, et al. Mass spectrometry-based hepcidin measurements in serum and urine: analytical aspects and clinical implications. Clin Chem 2007;53(4):620–8.
22. Ganz T, Olbina G, Girelli D, et al. Immunoassay for human serum hepcidin. Blood 2008;112(10):4292–7.

23. Velasco G, Cal S, Quesada V, et al. Matriptase-2, a membrane-bound mosaic serine proteinase predominantly expressed in human liver and showing degrading activity against extracellular matrix proteins. J Biol Chem 2002;277(40): 37637–46.

24. Ramsay AJ, Hooper JD, Folgueras AR, et al. Matriptase-2 (TMPRSS6): a proteolytic regulator of iron homeostasis. Haematologica 2009;94(6):840–9.

25. Stirnberg M, Maurer E, Horstmeyer A, et al. Proteolytic processing of the serine protease matriptase-2: identification of the cleavage sites required for its autocatalytic release from the cell surface. Biochem J 2010;430(1):87–95.

26. Sanders AJ, Webb SL, Parr C, et al. The type II transmembrane serine protease, matriptase-2: possible links to cancer? Anticancer Agents Med Chem 2010; 10(1):64–9.

27. Folgueras AR, de Lara FM, Pendas AM, et al. Membrane-bound serine protease matriptase-2 (Tmprss6) is an essential regulator of iron homeostasis. Blood 2008;112(6):2539–45.

28. Meynard D, Babitt JL, Lin HY. The liver: conductor of systemic iron balance. Blood 2014;123(2):168–76.

29. Kautz L, Meynard D, Monnier A, et al. Iron regulates phosphorylation of Smad1/5/8 and gene expression of Bmp6, Smad7, Id1, and Atoh8 in the mouse liver. Blood 2008;112(4):1503–9.

30. Andriopoulos B Jr, Corradini E, Xia Y, et al. BMP6 is a key endogenous regulator of hepcidin expression and iron metabolism. Nat Genet 2009;41(4):482–7.

31. Meynard D, Kautz L, Darnaud V, et al. Lack of the bone morphogenetic protein BMP6 induces massive iron overload. Nat Genet 2009;41(4):478–81.

32. Silvestri L, Pagani A, Nai A, et al. The serine protease matriptase-2 (TMPRSS6) inhibits hepcidin activation by cleaving membrane hemojuvelin. Cell Metab 2008;8(6):502–11.

33. Babitt JL, Huang FW, Wrighting DM, et al. Bone morphogenetic protein signaling by hemojuvelin regulates hepcidin expression. Nat Genet 2006; 38(5):531–9.

34. Papanikolaou G, Samuels ME, Ludwig EH, et al. Mutations in HFE2 cause iron overload in chromosome 1q-linked juvenile hemochromatosis. Nat Genet 2004;36(1):77–82.

35. Truksa J, Gelbart T, Peng H, et al. Suppression of the hepcidin-encoding gene Hamp permits iron overload in mice lacking both hemojuvelin and matriptase-2/TMPRSS6. Br J Haematol 2009;147(4):571–81.

36. Finberg KE, Whittlesey RL, Fleming MD, et al. Down-regulation of Bmp/Smad signaling by Tmprss6 is required for maintenance of systemic iron homeostasis. Blood 2010;115(18):3817–26.

37. Lenoir A, Deschemin JC, Kautz L, et al. Iron-deficiency anemia from matriptase-2 inactivation is dependent on the presence of functional Bmp6. Blood 2011; 117(2):647–50.

38. Lakhal S, Schodel J, Townsend AR, et al. Regulation of type II transmembrane serine proteinase TMPRSS6 by hypoxia-inducible factors: new link between hypoxia signaling and iron homeostasis. J Biol Chem 2011;286(6):4090–7.

39. Maurer E, Gutschow M, Stirnberg M. Matriptase-2 (TMPRSS6) is directly up-regulated by hypoxia inducible factor-1: identification of a hypoxia-responsive element in the TMPRSS6 promoter region. Biol Chem 2012;393(6):535–40.

40. Zhang AS, Anderson SA, Wang J, et al. Suppression of hepatic hepcidin expression in response to acute iron deprivation is associated with an increase of matriptase-2 protein. Blood 2011;117(5):1687–99.

41. Meynard D, Vaja V, Sun CC, et al. Regulation of TMPRSS6 by BMP6 and iron in human cells and mice. Blood 2011;118(3):747–56.
42. Meynard D, Sun CC, Wu Q, et al. Inflammation regulates TMPRSS6 expression via STAT5. PLoS One 2013;8(12):e82127.
43. Silvestri L, Guillem F, Pagani A, et al. Molecular mechanisms of the defective hepcidin inhibition in TMPRSS6 mutations associated with iron-refractory iron deficiency anemia. Blood 2009;113(22):5605–8.
44. Edison ES, Athiyarath R, Rajasekar T, et al. A novel splice site mutation c.2278 (-1) G>C in the TMPRSS6 gene causes deletion of the substrate binding site of the serine protease resulting in refractory iron deficiency anaemia. Br J Haematol 2009;147(5):766–9.
45. Tchou I, Diepold M, Pilotto PA, et al. Haematologic data, iron parameters and molecular findings in two new cases of iron-refractory iron deficiency anaemia. Eur J Haematol 2009;83(6):595–602.
46. De Falco L, Totaro F, Nai A, et al. Novel TMPRSS6 mutations associated with iron-refractory iron deficiency anemia (IRIDA). Hum Mutat 2010;31(5): E1390–405.
47. Altamura S, D'Alessio F, Selle B, et al. A novel TMPRSS6 mutation that prevents protease auto-activation causes IRIDA. Biochem J 2010;431(3):363–71.
48. Beutler E, Van Geet C, te Loo DM, et al. Polymorphisms and mutations of human TMPRSS6 in iron deficiency anemia. Blood Cells Mol Dis 2010;44(1):16–21.
49. Cuijpers ML, Wiegerinck ET, Brouwer R, et al. Iron deficiency anaemia due to a matriptase-2 mutation. Ned Tijdschr Geneeskd 2010;154:A1038 [in Dutch].
50. Choi HS, Yang HR, Song SH, et al. A novel mutation Gly603Arg of TMPRSS6 in a Korean female with iron-refractory iron deficiency anemia. Pediatr Blood Cancer 2012;58(4):640–2.
51. Guillem F, Kannengiesser C, Oudin C, et al. Inactive matriptase-2 mutants found in IRIDA patients still repress hepcidin in a transfection assay despite having lost their serine protease activity. Hum Mutat 2012;33(9):1388–96.
52. Pellegrino RM, Coutinho M, D'Ascola D, et al. Two novel mutations in the TMPRSS6 gene associated with iron-refractory iron-deficiency anaemia (IRIDA) and partial expression in the heterozygous form. Br J Haematol 2012;158(5): 668–72.
53. Jaspers A, Caers J, Le Gac G, et al. A novel mutation in the CUB sequence of matriptase-2 (TMPRSS6) is implicated in iron-resistant iron deficiency anaemia (IRIDA). Br J Haematol 2013;160(4):564–5.
54. Khuong-Quang DA, Schwartzentruber J, Westerman M, et al. Iron refractory iron deficiency anemia: presentation with hyperferritinemia and response to oral iron therapy. Pediatrics 2013;131(2):e620–5.
55. Yimaz Keskin E, Sal E, de Falco L, et al. Is the acronym IRIDA acceptable for slow responders to iron in the presence of TMPRSS6 mutations? Turk J Pediatr 2013;55(5):479–84.
56. Lehmberg K, Grosse R, Muckenthaler MU, et al. Administration of recombinant erythropoietin alone does not improve the phenotype in iron refractory iron deficiency anemia patients. Ann Hematol 2013;92(3):387–94.
57. Nai A, Pagani A, Silvestri L, et al. Increased susceptibility to iron deficiency of Tmprss6-haploinsufficient mice. Blood 2010;116(5):851–2.
58. The International HapMap Consortium. The international HapMap project. Nature 2003;426(6968):789–96.
59. The 1000 Genomes Project Consortium. An integrated map of genetic variation from 1,092 human genomes. Nature 2012;491(7422):56–65.

60. Benyamin B, McRae AF, Zhu G, et al. Variants in TF and HFE explain approximately 40% of genetic variation in serum-transferrin levels. Am J Hum Genet 2009;84(1):60–5.
61. Benyamin B, Ferreira MA, Willemsen G, et al. Common variants in TMPRSS6 are associated with iron status and erythrocyte volume. Nat Genet 2009;41(11): 1173–5.
62. Chambers JC, Zhang W, Li Y, et al. Genome-wide association study identifies variants in TMPRSS6 associated with hemoglobin levels. Nat Genet 2009; 41(11):1170–2.
63. Ganesh SK, Zakai NA, van Rooij FJ, et al. Multiple loci influence erythrocyte phenotypes in the CHARGE Consortium. Nat Genet 2009;41(11):1191–8.
64. Soranzo N, Spector TD, Mangino M, et al. A genome-wide meta-analysis identifies 22 loci associated with eight hematological parameters in the HaemGen consortium. Nat Genet 2009;41(11):1182–90.
65. Tanaka T, Roy CN, Yao W, et al. A genome-wide association analysis of serum iron concentrations. Blood 2010;115(1):94–6.
66. Nai A, Pagani A, Silvestri L, et al. TMPRSS6 rs855791 modulates hepcidin transcription in vitro and serum hepcidin levels in normal individuals. Blood 2011; 118(16):4459–62.
67. Traglia M, Girelli D, Biino G, et al. Association of HFE and TMPRSS6 genetic variants with iron and erythrocyte parameters is only in part dependent on serum hepcidin concentrations. J Med Genet 2011;48(9):629–34.
68. Galesloot TE, Geurts-Moespot AJ, den Heijer M, et al. Associations of common variants in HFE and TMPRSS6 with iron parameters are independent of serum hepcidin in a general population: a replication study. J Med Genet 2013; 50(9):593–8.
69. Finberg KE, Whittlesey RL, Andrews NC. Tmprss6 is a genetic modifier of the Hfe-hemochromatosis phenotype in mice. Blood 2011;117(17):4590–9.
70. Nai A, Pagani A, Mandelli G, et al. Deletion of TMPRSS6 attenuates the phenotype in a mouse model of beta-thalassemia. Blood 2012;119(21):5021–9.
71. Valenti L, Fracanzani AL, Rametta R, et al. Effect of the A736V TMPRSS6 polymorphism on the penetrance and clinical expression of hereditary hemochromatosis. J Hepatol 2012;57(6):1319–25.
72. Pelusi S, Girelli D, Rametta R, et al. The A736V TMPRSS6 polymorphism influences hepcidin and iron metabolism in chronic hemodialysis patients: TMPRSS6 and hepcidin in hemodialysis. BMC Nephrol 2013;14:48.
73. Valenti L, Rametta R, Dongiovanni P, et al. The A736V TMPRSS6 polymorphism influences hepatic iron overload in nonalcoholic fatty liver disease. PLoS One 2012;7(11):e48804.
74. Camaschella C. How I manage patients with atypical microcytic anaemia. Br J Haematol 2013;160(1):12–24.
75. Cau M, Galanello R, Giagu N, et al. Responsiveness to oral iron and ascorbic acid in a patient with IRIDA. Blood Cells Mol Dis 2012;48(2):121–3.
76. Nie N, Shi J, Shao Y, et al. A novel tri-allelic mutation of TMPRSS6 in iron-refractory iron deficiency anaemia with response to glucocorticoid. Br J Haematol 2014. [Epub ahead of print].
77. Gross SJ, Stuart MJ, Swender PT, et al. Malabsorption of iron in children with iron deficiency. J Pediatr 1976;88(5):795–9.
78. Molla AM, Verpoorten C, Eggermont E. The intestinal mucosa of children with iron deficiency. Acta Paediatr Belg 1973;27(1):5–12.

Sideroblastic Anemia
Diagnosis and Management

Sylvia S. Bottomley, MD[a],*, Mark D. Fleming, MD, DPhil[b]

KEYWORDS

- Sideroblastic anemia • Myelodysplastic syndrome • Ring sideroblasts
- Iron overload • Heme synthesis • Iron-sulfur clusters
- Mitochondrial iron metabolism • Ineffective erythropoiesis

KEY POINTS

- Sideroblastic anemias are diverse metabolic diseases of the erythroid cell.
- The presence of bone marrow ring sideroblasts is the diagnostic feature of all sideroblastic anemias.
- The disease course can usually be predicted when the underlying cause is identified.
- Systemic iron overload that occurs in the common sideroblastic anemias is mediated by ineffective erythropoiesis and leads to morbidity and reduced survival if untreated.

GENERAL OVERVIEW

When first defined 50 years ago, sideroblastic anemia (SA) was already recognized to occur in heterogeneous settings, including as familial or acquired disease.[1] The spectrum of SA has since become considerably expanded with respect to distinct clinical phenotypes as well as discrete causes.[2] The singular feature that typifies all forms of SA and is required for initial diagnosis is the presence of telltale ring sideroblasts in the bone marrow aspirate smear. These erythroblasts contain numerous coarse Prussian blue–positive granules, characteristically appearing in a perinuclear distribution (**Fig. 1**A), which represent pathologic deposits of iron in mitochondria (see **Fig. 1**B).

The magnitude of the quantity of iron used by the erythron to make hemoglobin is well appreciated. Hemoglobin contains nearly 80% of the body heme and therein more than two-thirds of the body iron. Heme is assembled from iron and protoporphyrin

a Department of Medicine, University of Oklahoma College of Medicine, 755 Research Park, Suite 427, Oklahoma City, OK 73104, USA; b Department of Pathology, Boston Children's Hospital, Harvard Medical School, 300 Longwood Avenue, Bader 124.1, Boston, MA 02115, USA
* Corresponding author.
E-mail address: sylvia-bottomley@ouhsc.edu

Hematol Oncol Clin N Am 28 (2014) 653–670
http://dx.doi.org/10.1016/j.hoc.2014.04.008
0889-8588/14/$ – see front matter © 2014 Elsevier Inc. All rights reserved.

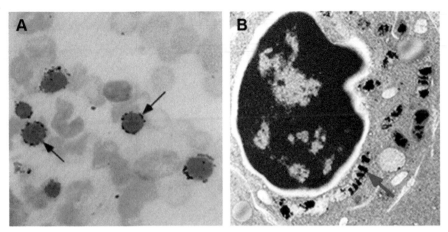

Fig. 1. Bone marrow with ring sideroblasts. (*A*) Bone marrow aspirate stained with Prussian blue, showing red cell precursors with numerous iron-positive granules (*arrows*). (*B*) Electron micrograph of an erythroblast with iron-laden (electron-dense deposits) mitochondria (*arrow*) clustered near the nucleus.

IX in the mitochondrion by ferrochelatase (FECH). However, iron imported into mitochondria is also required to generate iron-sulfur (Fe-S) clusters, which themselves participate as essential prosthetic groups in proteins regulating cellular iron uptake, heme synthesis, and iron storage, including iron regulatory protein 1 (IRP1) and FECH itself.[3]

General concepts regarding the pathogenesis of the SAs have emerged from discoveries of the genetic defects underlying various congenital SAs (CSAs). Based on our current knowledge, the unique pathology can be primarily linked to abnormalities in the heme biosynthesis and Fe-S biogenesis pathways as well as to defects in the translation of mitochondrially encoded proteins (**Fig. 2**). Nevertheless, in most instances, our understanding of the downstream events that lead to ring sideroblast formation and anemia is severely lacking. Importantly, body iron metabolism is also strikingly altered in the common SAs, in that the associated ineffective erythropoiesis elicits a systemic iron overload state, which often influences clinical features as well as prognosis, as discussed later.

DIAGNOSIS

The SAs can be divided into CSA and acquired forms. Although they are inherited, the CSAs may not present at birth, and sometimes may not be recognized until adulthood. Because of certain distinctive treatments and considerably different prognoses, it is particularly important to distinguish later-onset CSA from an acquired SA. As summarized later, the recognition of the specific diagnosis relies on characteristics of the anemia (eg, microcytic, normocytic, or macrocytic), the age of clinical onset, associated syndromic features, and, increasingly, molecular genetic diagnostics (**Table 1**).

Nonsyndromic CSAs

X-linked SA (XLSA) is the most common CSA, constituting about 40% of cases.[4] It is often mild or asymptomatic and may be discovered only in young adulthood or even in later life; occasional severe cases have presented in infancy or childhood.[2] Rarely is it associated with an in utero (often lethal) phenotype.[5] Not uncommonly, it is seen in

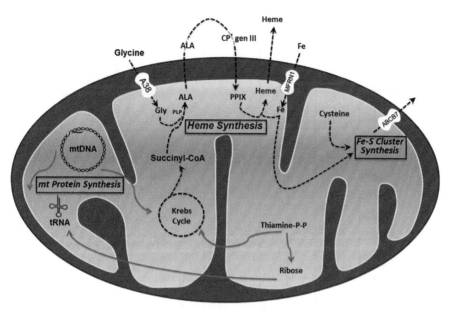

Fig. 2. Mitochondrial pathways in the erythroblast affected by genetic defects of CSAs. A38, SLC25A38; ABCB7, mitochondrial transporter for cytosolic Fe-S cluster protein maturation; ALA, 5-aminlevulinic acid; CoA, coenzyme A; CP'gen III, coproporphyrinogen III; Fe, iron; Gly, glycine; MFRN1, mitoferrin 1; mt, mitochondrial; PLP, pyridoxal 5'-phosphate; PPIX, protoporphyrin IX; thiamine-P-P, thiamine pyrophosphate; tRNA, transfer RNA.

women as a result of acquired skewed X chromosome inactivation in hematopoietic tissue, which occurs with advancing age.[6] Skewed constitutional X chromosome inactivation to account for disease expression in females in childhood is exceptional.

Mutations in ALAS2, the first and rate-controlling enzyme of heme synthesis, cause XLSA. More than 80 distinct mutations have been identified in more than 120 unrelated kindreds or probands.[2,3,7–9] About one-fifth of the mutations have occurred in more than 1 family, and nearly one-third of probands are female. Most of the mutations are missense alleles. Rare stop or frame shift alleles are viable only in females. Recently, several mutations affecting a GATA transcription factor binding site in intron 1 of the *ALAS2* gene were discovered.[8,9] These heterogeneous molecular defects predict diverse effects on the function of the ALAS2 enzyme and in turn variable severity of anemia.[3,10]

An autosomal recessive CSA caused by mutations in SLC25A38, accounting for about 15% of CSAs,[4] presents at birth or in early childhood as a severe, transfusion-dependent microcytic hypochromic anemia. The genetic defect involves the erythroid-specific mitochondrial inner membrane carrier protein SLC25A38, predicted to be an amino acid transporter required to import the ALAS2 substrate glycine, or possibly exchanging glycine for ALA, across the inner mitochondrial membrane in the initial steps of heme synthesis.[11] Among 31 patients so far reported, mutations are heterogeneous and include missense as well as nonsense and splicing errors, with one-fourth of them being recurrent in unrelated families.[7,11,12] Most mutations seem to be severe or complete loss-of-function mutations. Because of its autosomal location, this anemia is more likely seen in children of consanguineous parentage.

A single case of a microcytic hypochromic transfusion-dependent SA presenting in midlife has been attributed to a homozygous splice site mutation in the glutaredoxin 5

Table 1
Classification, genetic, and clinical features of the SAs

SA Class	Mutations Identified		Inheritance	Clinical Onset	Severity of Anemia	Mean Corpuscular Volume	Red Blood Cell Protoporphyrin	Associated Abnormalities
	Gene	Protein						
CSA								
Nonsyndromic CSA								
X-linked (XLSA)	*ALAS2*	ALAS2	X-linked	Variable	Mild to severe	↓[c]	N/↓	Iron overload
SLC25A38 deficiency	*SLC25A38*	mt transporter SLC25A38	AR	Childhood	Severe	↓	N/↓	Iron overload
Glutaredoxin 5 deficiency[a]	*GLRX5*	Glutaredoxin 5	AR	Adulthood	Mild to severe	↓	Not reported	Iron overload
Erythropoietic protoporphyria (EPP)[b]	*FECH*	FECH	AR	Usually childhood	Mild	↓	Marked ↑	Acute photosensitivity
Syndromic CSA								
X-linked with ataxia (XLSA/A)	*ABCB7*	mt transporter ABCB7	X-linked	Childhood	Mild to moderate	↓	↑	Incoordination, delayed motor development
SA, B-cell immunodeficiency, fevers and developmental delay (SIFD)	Unknown	Unknown	AR	Infancy	Severe	↓	Not reported	Iron overload, CNS derangements, deafness, cardiomyopathy
Pearson marrow-pancreas syndrome	*mtDNA*	Mitochondrial tRNAs	Sporadic/maternal	Early childhood	Severe	↑	↑	Metabolic acidosis, exocrine pancreatic insufficiency, hepatic/renal failure

	Gene	Protein/function	Inheritance	Age of onset	Anemia severity			Other features
Myopathy, lactic acidosis, and SA (MLASA)	PUS1/ YARS2	Pseudouridine synthase 1/mt tyrosyl tRNA synthetase	AR	Childhood	Mild to severe	N/↑	Not reported	Myopathy, lactic acidosis/ cardiomyopathy ±
Thiamine-responsive megaloblastic anemia (TRMA)	SLC19A2	Thiamine transporter	AR	Childhood	Severe	↑	N/↑	Non-type I diabetes, sensorineural deafness
Syndromic/ nonsyndromic SA of unknown cause	Unknown	Unknown	Varied	Variable	Variable	Variable	Variable	± diverse
Acquired SA								
Clonal/neoplastic								
RARS	SF3B1	Core component of RNA spliceosome	—	Adulthood	Mild to severe	N/↑	↑	Iron overload
RARS-T			—		Moderate	N/↑	Not reported	Thrombocytosis
RCMD-RS			—		Mild to severe	N/↑	Not reported	Cytopenias
Metabolic								
Alcoholism	—	—	—	Adulthood	Variable	N/↑	Variable	Nutritional/toxic effects of alcohol
Drug-induced	—	—	—	Adulthood	Variable	Variable	Variable	None
Copper deficiency (zinc toxicity)	—	—	—	Any age	Variable	N/↑	↑	Neurologic deficits, neutropenia
Hypothermia	—	—	—	3 adults reported	Mild to moderate	N/↑	Not reported	CNS features

Abbreviations: AR, autosomal recessive; CNS, central nervous system; mt, mitochondrial; N, normal; RARS, refractory anemia with ring sideroblasts; RARS-T, RARS with thrombocytosis; RCMD-RS, refractory cytopenia with multilineage dysplasia and ring sideroblasts; tRNA, transfer RNA; ↓, decreased; ↑, increased.

a Described in only 1 patient.
b Ring sideroblasts shown in 10 cases.
c Typically normal or increased in females expressing XLSA.

(*GLRX5*) gene.[13] In this instructive case, it could be shown that GLRX5 deficiency severely impairs Fe-S cluster biogenesis, which reduces ALAS2 translation through increased iron-responsive element binding activity of IRP1 lacking the Fe-S cluster, as well as the integrity of FECH deprived of its Fe-S cluster.[14]

Ring sideroblasts have been documented in only 10 patients with erythropoietic protoporphyria (EPP),[15] a disorder characterized by marked deficiency of FECH.[16] Mild anemia is observed in most patients,[17] but it is uncertain that EPP consistently results in a CSA marrow phenotype.

The clinical laboratory clue for each of the nonsyndromic CSAs is erythrocyte microcytosis and hypochromia (reduced mean corpuscular volume [MCV] and mean corpuscular hemoglobin), along with an increased red cell distribution width (RDW) and absence of evidence for common causes of microcytic anemia such as iron deficiency and thalassemia. An important exception to this characteristic is that most females expressing XLSA have a normal or increased MCV. In severely affected females, erythroid cells with a nonfunctional ALAS2 enzyme presumably do not develop into viable erythrocytes, so that the patients' circulating red cells represent progeny of the residual normal clone released from marrow at an accelerated rate in response to the anemia. Some females with milder anemia have a biphasic red cell volume histogram characterized by populations of normocytic and microcytic cells. Nonanemic female carriers of this trait may or may not have a small microcytic circulating erythrocyte population, but when present, may suggest the correct diagnosis in a related male proband. The morphologic features of the anemia in individuals affected by SLC25A38 mutations are indistinguishable from males with XLSA. Nonetheless, it is exceptional for XLSA to present in early childhood, and, consequently, mutations in SLC25A38 should be excluded in all individuals presenting with microcytic CSA in infancy or early childhood. As is true of all CSAs, the definitive diagnosis rests on showing a genetic defect by mutational analysis (see **Table 1**).

Syndromic CSAs

The presence of nonhematologic manifestations distinguishes the syndromic CSAs from the nonsyndromic CSAs. Sometimes, the associated features may be subtle or not yet fully manifest at the time of presentation, making recognition on clinical grounds elusive.

XLSA with ataxia (XLSA/A), described in 4 kindreds to date, is characterized by mild to moderate microcytic SA accompanied by neurologic deficits of delayed motor and cognitive development, incoordination, and cerebellar hypoplasia.[18,19] Female carriers of XLSA/A show mild hematologic abnormalities, including an increased RDW and occasional peripheral blood siderocytes, but no neurologic manifestations. XLSA/A is caused by mutations in the mitochondrial adenosine triphosphate–binding cassette transporter ABCB7, which is postulated to participate in the export of Fe-S clusters generated in mitochondria for assembly of cytosolic Fe-S cluster-containing proteins.[20] Like mutations in GLRX5, it is presumed that ABCB7 dysfunction disturbs cellular and mitochondrial iron metabolism through its effects on IRP1, among other proteins.

The syndrome of CSA, B-cell immunodeficiency, periodic fevers, and developmental delay (SIFD) presents in infancy and is also variably associated with central nervous system (CNS) abnormalities, sensorineural hearing loss, and cardiomyopathy.[21] The anemia is microcytic and severe, often requiring chronic transfusion or stem cell transplantation. Inheritance is autosomal recessive.

The Pearson marrow-pancreas syndrome generally presents within the first 6 months of life with failure to thrive, anemia ± other cytopenias, metabolic acidosis, and exocrine pancreatic insufficiency; hepatic and renal failure are also common.[22] Absence of the metabolic derangements initially may result in oversight of the syndrome, particularly when ring sideroblasts are rare or when there is a marked erythroid hypoplasia, in which case the disorder may be mistaken for Diamond-Blackfan anemia.[23,24] The anemia tends to be severe and is most often macrocytic. In the bone marrow, there is striking vacuolization of erythroid and myeloid progenitors.[25] In skeletal muscle there are marked abnormalities in mitochondrial ultrastructure, most characteristically parking lot inclusions in mitochondria, which represent linear arrays of cristae. Deletions (most often of 4977 bp, which is common to many mitochondrial cytopathies), rearrangements, or duplications of mitochondrial DNA (mtDNA) are diagnostic.[26] The heteroplasmy of mtDNA at the cellular and organ levels accounts for the high variability of affected tissues, which may even evolve over time. There is no single common deleted region in all patients. Instead, it seems that 1 or several mitochondrially encoded transfer RNAs (tRNA) are deleted in nearly all cases, and would be expected to lead to a global defect in mitochondrial protein translation. As in several other forms of CSA, the mechanism for the mitochondrial iron accumulation is not understood.

The central role of mitochondrial tRNAs and mitochondrial translation in the pathogenesis of several of the syndromic CSAs is reinforced by mitochondrial myopathy, lactic acidosis, and SA (MLASA), which is an autosomal recessive disorder encountered in infancy, childhood, or adolescence. The cardinal clinical findings are skeletal muscle weakness, variably severe normocytic anemia, and lactic acidosis. Vacuolization of marrow progenitors and ultrastructural findings on skeletal muscle electron microscopy are indistinguishable from Pearson marrow-pancreas syndrome. Mutations in 2 genes result in the MLASA phenotype. Pseudouridine synthase 1 (PUS1) posttranscriptionally modifies cytosolic as well as mitochondrial tRNAs by converting uridine to pseudouridine, stabilizing the tRNA secondary structure.[27–29] Mitochondrial tyrosyl tRNA synthetase (YARS2) charges the mitochondrially encoded tyrosine tRNA with its cognate amino acid.[29,30] Missense and nonsense mutations in either protein presumptively lead to decreased mitochondrial protein synthesis and respiratory chain dysfunction, but how these mitochondrial protein deficiencies cause mitochondrial iron accumulation and anemia is unclear.

Thiamine-responsive megaloblastic anemia (TRMA) syndrome typically manifests as a triad of megaloblastic anemia, non–type I diabetes mellitus, and sensorineural deafness between infancy and adolescence.[31] The macrocytic anemia is associated with variable neutropenia and thrombocytopenia and megaloblastic changes. The molecular diagnosis is established by biallelic mutations in the *SLC19A2* gene, which encodes a high-affinity thiamine transporter. Most mutations are nonsense or frameshift mutations leading to complete loss-of-function alleles, but increasingly, missense alleles have been identified in individuals with less overt TRMA phenotypes.[32] The macrocytic megaloblastic anemia is considered to result from defective nucleic acid synthesis attributed to cellular thiamine deficiency.[33] The ring sideroblasts are hypothesized to relate to the role of thiamine in the production of succinyl-coenzyme A, a substrate of ALAS.[34]

Undefined CSAs

Up to 40% of CSA cases are molecularly unexplained.[4,7,35] In these cases, autosomal recessive as well as X-linked defects are possible and may be shown in previously identified genes causing the phenotype with other approaches of mutational analysis. Alternatively, within the presently understood pathophysiologic framework of iron homeostasis in the erythroid cell, novel genes involving heme or Fe-S cluster production, as well as mitochondrial proteins that affect iron processing or utilization, may be discovered.

Acquired Clonal SAs

This most common SA encountered in clinical practice develops insidiously in middle-aged and older individuals. It may be discovered during a routine examination or in association with an unrelated complaint. The anemia is usually of moderate severity, normocytic or macrocytic, but dimorphic because of the presence of a hypochromic erythrocyte population on the blood smear.[36]

The disorder is a bone marrow stem cell disorder and classified within the rubric of myelodysplastic syndromes (MDS) and myeloproliferative neoplasms. In the current World Health Organization classification of hematopoietic neoplasms, 3 variants are distinguished: refractory anemia with ring sideroblasts (RARS), RARS with thrombocytosis (RARS-T), and refractory cytopenia with multilineage dysplasia and ring sideroblasts (RCMD-RS).[37] Classification into each of these forms, as the names indicate, depends on the presence or absence of dysplasia within the nonerythroid marrow lineages as well as the clinical absence or presence of thrombocytosis. As is described later, there is increasing molecular evidence that these disorders are on a continuous phenotypic spectrum that is related to primary driver somatic mutations in a restricted class of genes, on which secondary mutations supervene to modify the morphologic and clinical phenotype.

In early work focusing on heme biosynthesis no consistent defects in protoporphyrin synthesis in marrow cells were found.[2] A somatic ALAS2 mutation was identified in only 1 case.[38] However, a constant feature is mild to moderate increase of erythrocyte protoporphyrin, and impaired marrow FECH activity was observed in about one-half of patients studied.[2] Uncommonly, clinical or biochemical features resemble EPP,[2,39] which may be explained by a likely acquired deletion of an FECH allele caused by a cytogenetic abnormality of the clonal disorder.[40]

Subsequently, intraclonal heterogeneity of the erythroblast phenotype (ie, a variable amount of mitochondrial iron overload evident from cell to cell) had suggested a heteroplasmic state caused by a mitochondrial defect(s). Extensive analysis of mtDNA in patients with RARS as well as other MDS forms showed a wide spectrum of heteroplasmic mutations across the mitochondrial genome in approximately one-half of cases.[41] Although their functional importance overall remains unclear, some mutations may affect mitochondrial iron metabolism (eg, if they affect cytochrome oxidase).[42]

In recent years, mutations in protein constituents of the spliceosome, which mediates maturation of primary mRNA transcripts into mature mRNAs lacking introns, have been recognized as being common in MDS. Specifically, acquired heterozygous missense alleles of the SF3B1 (splicing factor 3B, subunit 1) component of the splicing machinery are present in up to 85% of patients with RARS, RARS-T, and RCMD-RS.[43–47] The presence of multiple specific recurrent alleles localized to a restricted portion of the SF3B1 protein suggests that these mutations are not loss-of-function alleles, but rather gain-of-function variants or mutations that affect the function of the protein in an otherwise distinctive manner. In cases lacking an SF3B1 mutation, other spliceosome components, particularly SRSF2 or ZRSR2, are commonly mutated. Among the myriad of genes whose splicing and expression may be altered by mutations in the spliceosome, there is evidence to suggest that changes in ABCB7 expression may be the downstream mechanism(s) leading to the dysregulated iron metabolism and sideroblastic phenotype.[48,49]

The diagnosis of MDS with ring sideroblasts must be established by exclusion of other causes of SA. These conditions are rare, if they occur at all, in children and adults less than 40 years of age, in whom a congenital basis, and less likely a metabolic cause (see later discussion), should be considered. Moreover, because the hemato-logic phenotype of females expressing XLSA is indistinguishable from RARS, analysis of the *ALAS2* gene for mutations should be entertained in them.[50,51]

Acquired Metabolic SAs

Exposure to ethanol and certain drugs, as well as acquired copper deficiency, may lead to an SA with features that overlap with those of the congenital or acquired clonal forms. In these instances, the anemia is fully reversible when the offending factor is removed.

Ethanol, by disrupting heme synthesis, suppressing erythroid colony formation, and likely inhibiting mitochondrial protein synthesis, contributes to the usual multifactorial anemia associated with alcoholism.[2,3] The ring sideroblast abnormality is noted in up to one-third of anemic alcoholic patients and most characteristically in the presence of malnutrition and folate deficiency.[52,53] The MCV is normal or increased; dimorphic erythrocytes are common, and siderocytes may be present on the blood smear. A highly suggestive finding in bone marrow is vacuolization of pronormoblasts.

Although isoniazid and chloramphenicol have been the prototypical drugs that pro-duce an SA,[2] a series of other agents have been implicated and include cycloserine, pyrazinamide, linezolid, fusidic acid, busulfan, melphalan, penicillamine, and triethyle-netetramine dihydrochloride. Many antituberculosis drugs interfere with vitamin B_6 metabolism and impair heme synthesis.[2,54] Linezolid, a more recently used antibiotic, induces the ring sideroblast abnormality,[55,56] and its toxicity resembles that of chlor-amphenicol because it also inhibits mitochondrial protein synthesis although by a different mechanism.[57] The association with the other drugs was reported in single or in a few patients, and their toxicity in the erythron is not characterized.

Nutritional copper deficiency occurs when the metal is omitted in parenteral feed-ings, in malabsorption states, and after gastrointestinal resections.[2,3,58,59] Another cause is prolonged ingestion of zinc (eg, in zinc supplements, zinc-containing denture cream, coins).[2] Zinc induces metallothionein, resulting in sequestration of copper in the intestinal epithelium, and decreased absorption of copper in the gut.[60] Various neurologic manifestations, including CNS demyelination, peripheral neuropathy, optic neuropathy, and most often myeloneuropathy, are usually, if not invariably, present and, in time, become irreversible.[58,61] The anemia may be severe, the MCV is normal or increased, and neutropenia is frequent. Low serum copper and ceruloplasmin levels confirm the diagnosis.

DISEASE COURSES AND TREATMENT OPTIONS

The clinical courses of these heterogeneous disorders are highly dependent on the un-derlying cause as well as on the supportive care that the patient receives, particularly if the disease is severe.

Nonsyndromic CSA

In XLS, the anemia is usually mild to moderate in severity and remains so at the set point determined by the mutation-induced functional impairment of the ALAS2 enzyme. In up to two-thirds of cases, the anemia responds to the essential cofactor of ALAS in the form of pyridoxine supplements by enhancing the function of some ALAS2 mutants. On average, the hemoglobin level normalizes in about one-third of re-sponders. Uncommonly, severe anemia that is unresponsive to pyridoxine dictates transfusion dependence, with attendant accentuation of iron overload. This finding has also been observed in females expressing XLSA caused by severe ALAS2 mutations and progressive inactivation of the normal X chromosome with advancing age.

Patients with the uniformly severe anemia caused by SLC25A38 defects require regular transfusions lifelong. Hematopoietic stem cell transplantation has been successful in 5 unreported cases. In the single patient with GLRX5 deficiency, transfusions were believed to worsen the anemia, which was partially reversed by iron chelation with deferoxamine.[13] The mild anemia associated with EPP requires no treatment, but the patients' lifelong course of variable photosensitivity may be abruptly complicated by progressive liver disease in ~2% of cases, requiring liver and/or bone marrow transplantation.[62]

Syndromic CSA

The clinical course in the XLSA/A syndrome is dominated by the nonhematologic features of neurologic changes and is dependent on supportive or rehabilitative services.

The severity and progressive nature of SIFD has led to early death from cardiac or multiorgan failure in 53% of cases.[21] Supportive treatment has included regular transfusions and immunoglobulin infusions in most patients. Hematopoietic stem cell transplantation was successful in one, correcting the anemia and immunodeficiency.

Similarly, about one-half of patients with Pearson marrow-pancreas syndrome succumb to the associated metabolic derangements.[23] The anemia improves in survivors or they develop Kearns-Sayre syndrome.

Patients with the MLASA syndromes have had unpredictable clinical courses. Manifestations at presentation have been highly variable, even within or between families with the same genetic variant,[30,63–67] and some patients with YARS2 defects have shown spontaneous improvement.[30] Severe disease, also manifesting cardiomyopathy, portended demise in 2 cases at ages 3 months and 18 years.[30] Many patients have survived into adulthood.

In the TRMA syndrome phenotypic variability from the outset influences the prognosis. Thiamine (vitamin B_1) is prescribed in pharmacologic doses and usually improves the anemia and the diabetes, although it has become ineffective in adulthood.[68]

Acquired Clonal SA

The natural history of the RARS and RARS-T variants is typically a stable, nonprogressive anemia of many years duration.[47,69,70] Transfusions may be necessary for symptomatic anemia, in particular at advanced age or in the presence of other comorbid conditions. Patients with RCMD-RS tend to have more severe anemia, have decreased survival, and ~5% evolve into acute leukemia.[70]

Various agents used in therapeutic trials for MDS, which have included the ring sideroblast variants, have been erythropoietin with or without granulocyte colony-stimulating factor and various drugs (eg, 5-azacytidine and decitabine, etanercept, antithymocyte globulin, thalidomide and lenalidomide, and valproic acid).[2,3] On average, major responses with improved erythropoiesis have been limited or less than 50%.

Splenectomy in SA

This operation has often been considered and occasionally performed in patients with CSA with severe anemia and significant splenomegaly. Because this procedure is invariably complicated by postoperative thromboembolic disease and often a fatal outcome,[71–75] it should be considered contraindicated. Factors other than persistent thrombocytosis seem to play a role, and control of the platelet count and anticoagulant therapy are usually ineffective.

IRON OVERLOAD

Systemic iron overload, also termed erythropoietic hemochromatosis, develops to a variable degree in several forms of SA (see **Table 1**), but most prominently in CSA,[71,76,77] and it can significantly contribute to morbidity and mortality. Mild to moderate hepatosplenomegaly with preserved liver function is common. The iron deposition in liver is indistinguishable from hereditary hemochromatosis, being predominantly hepatocellular and periportal in nature.[2,78] In XLSA, the iron burden has not always correlated with the severity of the anemia and well-established cirrhosis may be discovered in the third or fourth decade even in patients not known to be anemic.[71,72,79,80] Hepatocellular carcinoma has developed in 2 reported cases.[81,82] In time, cardiac arrhythmias and congestive heart failure supervene. In children, growth and development may be impaired. The process is not HFE linked, although occasionally it may be accentuated by coinheritance of an HFE-hemochromatosis allele(s).

This form of iron overload is driven by the ineffective erythropoiesis so typical of SA (as well as thalassemia and congenital dyserythropoietic anemia) by mediating inappropriately increased intestinal absorption of iron[83] through suppression of the iron regulatory hormone hepcidin by an ill-defined mechanism.[84,85] Mediators such as GDF-15 (growth differentiating factor 15) and TWSG1 (twisted gastrulation) released from the ineffective erythron in the bone marrow have been postulated.[86,87] More recently, Erfe (erythroferrone) has been reported as the erythroid factor that represses hepcidin during increased erythropoietic activity.[88] However, the long sought after erythroid regulator of iron metabolism as first proposed by Finch[89] has not yet been definitively ascertained.

Repeated transfusions for severe anemia predictably add to the iron burden, because each unit of red cells delivers 200 to 300 mg of iron. Although transfusional iron overload may at least in part result in nonparenchymal distribution of the iron, it can significantly add to morbidity and affect survival.[69,90] As extensively shown in thalassemia, long ago, and, more recently, in limited studies in MDS, mortality can be improved with effective iron-chelation therapy.[91,92] Chelation limits nontransferrin-bound iron and labile iron pools in plasma and cells rapidly, whereas removal of iron stored in tissues is mobilized more slowly.[93] However, considerable debate persists regarding precise indications for chelation therapy in transfusional iron overload,[94] which also seemed to be reflected at least partly in the management variation of a large patient group.[95] Although the MDS Foundation's Working Group on Transfusional Iron Overload and other groups have developed consensus statements on the issue, data from prospective trials are desired.[96,97] Meanwhile, the decision regarding iron-chelation therapy in this setting is best based on current consensus statements as well as on a case-by-case basis.

Iron depletion is best performed by phlebotomy when the anemia is mild or moderate (ie, hemoglobin ≥ 9 g/dL), or when a patient with XLSA has responded to pyridoxine. After initial iron depletion, regular phlebotomies are continued for life to control iron reaccumulation. In patients with more severe anemia and who require regular red cell transfusions, iron chelation is used. The available agents in the United States for treatment of all transfusional iron overload disorders, including SA, are deferoxamine (Desferal, Novartis) for parenteral administration and deferasirox (Exjade, Novartis) as the oral preparation. A third chelating agent, deferiprone (Ferriprox, Apotex) is licensed for use in thalassemia with a second-line indication. Combinations of these drugs can be used in severe iron overload, although trials of such therapy in SA have not been performed and would be considered off label.

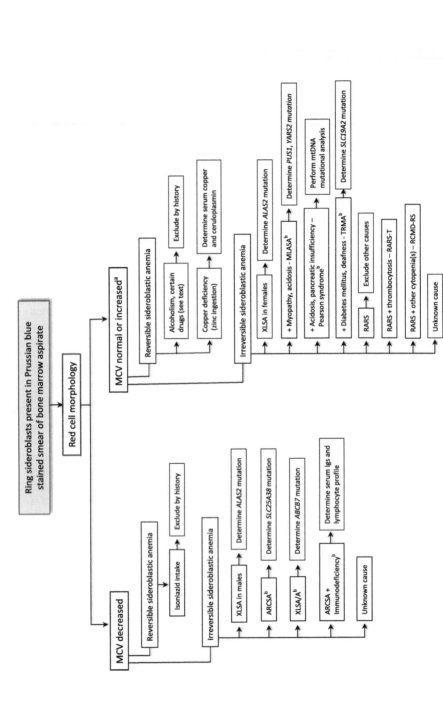

Fig. 3. Schema for diagnostic evaluation of patients with an SA. ARCSA, autosomal recessive CSA; Igs, immunoglobulins; TRMA, thiamine-responsive megaloblastic anemia. [a] Microcytic hypochromic red cells may be present in the blood smear in many, but not all, of these disorders. [b] Typically detected in infancy or childhood.

Anemia may improve after adequate iron removal.[2,98–100] An independent salutary effect of iron chelation on erythropoiesis was also implicated in some cases.

SUMMARY

Although SA is uncommon and some forms are rare, it should be considered in all adults and children/infants with unexplained anemia of any severity from history, clinical examination, and basic laboratory data. Certain clinical features are suggestive, such as history of chronic anemia; exposure to factors causing reversible SA; family history of anemia; presence of neurologic abnormalities; myopathy, lactic acidosis, immunodeficiency in children or young adults.

If the pathognomonic ring sideroblasts are evident on a Prussian blue stain of the bone marrow aspirate smear, a careful review of the patient's constellation of clinical findings and the erythrocyte indices and morphology aid in narrowing the differential diagnosis (**Fig. 3**, see **Table 1**). Erythrocyte morphology is most accurate before any transfusion, which can conceal the abnormalities (eg, a microcytosis and hypochromia). When the causative gene is known, mutation analysis provides the definitive diagnosis of a CSA. Some molecular genetic tests are available in several clinical laboratories, whereas others are available only in certain research laboratories. In cases of CSA in which the genetic cause is identified, a search for affected family members is advisable. In the common forms of SA, evaluation and monitoring for iron overload are indicated by biochemical testing (serum transferrin saturation and ferritin) and noninvasive assessment of parenchymal organ involvement by magnetic resonance imaging.

The principal treatments include withdrawal or correction of an identified reversible cause; if the anemia is microcytic, a therapeutic trial of pyridoxine supplement until the genetic cause can be determined (the vitamin is effective only in some cases of XLSA); red cell transfusion for symptomatic anemia; removal of excess iron by phlebotomy if anemia is milder and by use of iron chelation in patients with severe/transfusion-dependent anemia.

REFERENCES

1. Mollin DL. Sideroblasts and sideroblastic anaemia. Br J Haematol 1965;11: 41–8.
2. Bottomley SS. Sideroblastic anemias. In: Greer JP, Arbor DA, Glader B, et al, editors. Wintrobe's clinical hematology. 13th edition. Philadelphia: Lippincott Williams & Wilkins Health; 2014. p. 643–61.
3. Bottomley SS, Fleming MD. Sideroblastic anemias: molecular basis, pathophysiology and clinical aspects. In: Kadish KM, Smith KM, Guilard R, editors. Handbook of porphyrin science: with applications to chemistry, physics, materials science, engineering, biology and medicine, vol. 29. Hackensack (NJ): World Scientific Publishing; 2013. p. 43–87.
4. Bergmann AK, Campagna DR, McLoughlin SM, et al. Systematic molecular analysis of congenital sideroblastic anemia: evidence for genetic heterogeneity and identification of novel mutations. Pediatr Blood Cancer 2010;54(2):273–8.
5. Rose C, Oudin C, Fournier M, et al. A new ALAS2 mutation inducing a male lethal X-linked sideroblastic anemia [abstract]. Blood 2013;122(21):2199.
6. Busque I, Mio R, Mattioli J, et al. Non-random X-inactivation patterns in normal females: lyonization ratios vary with age. Blood 1996;88(1):59–65.
7. Liu G, Guo S, Kang H, et al. Mutation spectrum in Chinese patients affected by congenital sideroblastic anemia and a search for a genotype-phenotype relationship. Haematologica 2013;98(12):e158–60.

8. Campagna DR, deBie CI, Schmitz-Abe K, et al. X-linked sideroblastic anemia due to ALAS2 intron 1 enhancer element GATA-binding site mutations. Am J Hematol 2014;89(3):315–9.

9. Kaneko K, Furuyama K, Fujiwara T, et al. Identification of a novel erythroid-specific enhancer for the ALAS2 gene and its loss-of-function mutation which is associated with congenital sideroblastic anemia. Haematologica 2014; 99(2):252–61.

10. Astner I, Schulze JO, van den Heuvel J, et al. Crystal structure of 5-aminolevulinate synthase, the first enzyme of heme biosynthesis and its link to XLSA in humans. EMBO J 2005;24(18):3166–77.

11. Guernsey DL, Jiang H, Campagna D, et al. Mutations in mitochondrial carrier family gene SLC25A38 cause nonsyndromic autosomal-recessive congenital sideroblastic anemia. Nat Genet 2009;41(6):651–3.

12. Kannengiesser C, Sanchez M, Sweeney M, et al. Missense SLC25A38 variations play an important role in autosomal recessive hereditary sideroblastic anemia. Haematologica 2011;96(6):808–13.

13. Camaschella C, Campanella S, DeFalco L, et al. The human counterpart of zebrafish shiraz shows sideroblastic-like microcytic anemia and iron overload. Blood 2007;110(4):1353–8.

14. Ye H, Jeong SY, Ghosh MC, et al. Glutaredoxin 5 deficiency causes sideroblastic anemia by specifically impairing heme biosynthesis and depleting cytosolic iron in human erythroblasts. J Clin Invest 2010;120(5):1749–61.

15. Rademakers LH, Koningsberger JC, Sorber CW. Accumulation of iron in erythroblasts of patients with erythropoietic protoporphyria. Eur J Clin Invest 1993; 23(2):130–8.

16. Lecha M, Puy H, Deybach JC. Erythropoietic protoporphyria. Orphanet J Rare Dis 2009;4:19–28.

17. Holme SA, Worwood M, Anstey AV, et al. Erythropoiesis and iron metabolism in dominant erythropoietic protoporphyria. Blood 2007;110(12):4108–10.

18. Pagon RA, Bird TD, Detter JC, et al. Hereditary sideroblastic anaemia and ataxia: an X-linked recessive disorder. J Med Genet 1985;22(4):267–73.

19. D'Hooghe M, Selleslag D, Mortier G, et al. X-linked sideroblastic anaemia and ataxia: a new family with identification of a fourth ABCB7 gene mutation. Eur J Paediatr Neurol 2012;16(6):730–5.

20. Bekri S, Kispal G, Lange H, et al. Human ABCB7 transporter: gene structure and mutation causing X-linked sideroblastic anemia with ataxia with disruption of cytosolic iron-sulfur protein maturation. Blood 2000;96(9):3256–64.

21. Wiseman DH, May A, Jolles S, et al. A novel syndrome of congenital sideroblastic anemia, B-cell immunodeficiency, periodic fevers and developmental delay (SIFD). Blood 2013;122(1):112–23.

22. Rotig A, Cormier V, Blanch S, et al. Pearson's marrow-pancreas syndrome. A multisystem mitochondrial disorder of infancy. J Clin Invest 1990;86(5):1601–8.

23. Manea EM, Leverger G, Bellmann F, et al. Pearson syndrome in the neonatal period: two case reports and review of the literature. J Pediatr Hematol Oncol 2009;31(12):947–51.

24. Gagne KE, Ghazvinian R, Yuan D, et al. Pearson marrow pancreas syndrome in patients suspected to have diamond Blackfan anemia. Blood 2014. http://dx.doi.org/10.1182/blood-2014-01-545830.

25. Bader-Meunier B, Mielot F, Breton-Gorius J, et al. Hematologic involvement in mitochondrial cytopathies in childhood: a retrospective study of bone marrow smears. Pediatr Res 1999;46(2):158–62.

26. Rotig A, Gouargeron T, Chretien D, et al. Spectrum of mitochondrial DNA rearrangements in the Pearson marrow-pancreas syndrome. Hum Mol Genet 1995; 4(8):1327–30.

27. Bykhovskaya Y, Casas K, Mengesha E, et al. Missense mutation in pseudouridine synthase (PUS1) causes mitochondrial myopathy and sideroblastic anemia (MLASA). Am J Hum Genet 2004;74(6):1303–8.

28. Patton JR, Bykhovskaja Y, Mengesha E, et al. Mitochondrial myopathy and sideroblastic anemia (MLASA): missense mutation in the pseudouridine synthase (PUS1) gene is associated with the loss of tRNA pseudouridylation. J Biol Chem 2005;280(20):19823–8.

29. Suzuki T, Nagao A, Suzuki T. Human mitochondrial tRNAs: biogenesis, function, structural aspects, and diseases. Annu Rev Genet 2011;45:299–329.

30. Riley LG, Menezes MJ, Rudinger-Thirion J, et al. Phenotypic variability and identification of novel YARS2 mutations in YARS2 mitochondrial myopathy, lactic acidosis and sideroblastic anaemia. Orphanet J Rare Dis 2013;8:193–203.

31. Neufeld EJ, Fleming JC, Tartaglini E, et al. Thiamine-responsive megaloblastic anemia syndrome: a disorder of high-affinity thiamine transport. Blood Cells Mol Dis 2001;27(1):135–8.

32. Bergmann AK, Sahai I, Falcone JF, et al. Thiamine-responsive megaloblastic anemia: identification of novel compound heterozygotes and mutation update. J Pediatr 2009;155(6):888–92.

33. Boros LG, Steinkamp MP, Fleming JC, et al. Defective RNA ribose synthesis in fibroblasts from patients with thiamine-responsive megaloblastic anemia (TRMA). Blood 2003;102(10):3556–61.

34. Abboud MR, Alexander D, Najjar SS. Diabetes mellitus, thiamine-dependent megaloblastic anemia, and sensorineural deafness associated with deficiency alpha-ketoglutarate dehydrogenase deficiency. J Pediatr 1985;107(4):537–41.

35. Ducamp S, Kannengiesser C, Touati M, et al. Sideroblastic anemia: molecular analysis of the ALAS2 gene in a series of 29 probands and functional studies of 10 missense mutations. Hum Mutat 2011;32(6):590–7.

36. Kushner JP, Lee GR, Wintrobe MM, et al. Idiopathic refractory sideroblastic anemia. Clinical and laboratory investigation of 17 patients and review of the literature. Medicine 1971;50(3):139–59.

37. Swerdlow SH, Campo E, Harris NL, et al, World Health Organization. WHO classification of tumours of haematopoietic and lymphoid tissues. 4th edition. Lyon (France): International Agency for Research on Cancer; 2008.

38. May A, Al-Sabah AI, Lawless SL. Acquired sideroblastic anemia unresponsive to pyridoxine caused by a somatic mutation I ALA synthase 2 [abstract]. Blood 2005;106(11):988a–9a.

39. Bottomley SS, Muller-Eberhard U. Pathophysiology of heme synthesis. Semin Hematol 1988;25(4):282–302.

40. Sarkany RP, Ross G, Willis F. Acquired erythropoietic protoporphyria as a result of myelodysplasia causing loss of chromosome 18. Brit J Dermatol 2006;155(2): 464–6.

41. Wulfert M, Kupper AC, Tapprich C, et al. Analysis of mitochondrial DNA in 104 patients with myelodysplastic syndrome. Exp Hematol 2008;36(5):577–86.

42. Gattermann N, Retzlaff S, Wang YL, et al. Heteroplasmic point mutations of mitochondrial DNA affecting subunit 1 of cytochrome c oxidase in two patients with acquired idiopathic sideroblastic anemia. Blood 1997;90(12):4961–72.

43. Papaemmanuil E, Cazzola M, Boultwood J, et al. Somatic SF3B1 mutation in myelodysplasia with ring sideroblasts. N Engl J Med 2011;365(15):1384–95.

44. Patnaik MM, Lasho TM, Hodnefield JM, et al. SF3B1 mutations are prevalent in myelodysplastic syndromes with ring sideroblasts but do not hold independent prognostic value. Blood 2012;119(2):569–72.

45. Visconte V, Makishima H, Jankowska A, et al. SF3B1, a splicing factor is frequently mutated in refractory anemia with ring sideroblasts. Leukemia 2012;26(3):542–5.

46. Damm F, Kosmider O, Gelsi-Boyer V, et al. Mutations affecting mRNA splicing define distinct clinical phenotypes and correlate with patient outcome in myelodysplastic syndromes. Blood 2012;119(14):3211–8.

47. Broseus J, Alpermann T, Wulfert M, et al. Age, JAK2(V617F) and SF2B1 mutations are the main predicting factors for survival in refractory anaemia with ring sideroblasts and marked thrombocytosis. Leukemia 2013;27(9):1826–31.

48. Boultwood J, Pellagatti A, Nikpour M, et al. The role of the iron transporter ABCB7 in refractory anemia with ring sideroblasts. PLoS One 2008;3(4):e1970.

49. Nikpour M, Scharenberg C, Liu A, et al. The transporter ABCB7 is a mediator of the phenotype of acquired refractory anemia with ring sideroblasts. Leukemia 2013;27(4):889–96.

50. Bottomley SS, Wise PD, Wasson EG, et al. X-linked sideroblastic anemia in 10 female probands due to ALAS2 mutations and skewed X chromosome inactivation (Abstract). Am J Hum Genet 1998;63:A352.

51. Aivado M, Gattermann N, Rong A, et al. X-linked sideroblastic anemia associated with a novel ALAS2 mutation and unfortunate skewed X-chromosome inactivation patterns. Blood Cells Mol Dis 2006;37(1):40–5.

52. Eichner ER, Hillman RS. The evolution of anemia in alcoholic patients. Am J Med 1971;50(2):218–32.

53. Savage D, Lindenbaum J. Anemia in alcoholics. Medicine 1986;65(5):322–38.

54. Bottomley SS. Sideroblastic anaemia. In: Jacobs A, Worwood M, editors. Iron in biochemistry and medicine II. London: Academic Press; 1980. p. 363–92.

55. Saini N, Jacobson NO, Iha S, et al. The perils of not digging deep enough–uncovering a rare cause of acquired anemia. Am J Hematol 2012;87(4):413–6.

56. Willekens C, Dumezy F, Boyer T, et al. Linezolid induces ring sideroblasts. Haematologica 2013;98(11):e138–40.

57. Kloss P, Xiong L, Shinabanger DL, et al. Resistance mutations in 23 S rNA identify the site of action of the protein synthesis inhibitor linezolid in the ribosomal peptidyl transferase center. J Mol Biol 1999;294(1):93–101.

58. Kumar N. Copper deficiency myelopathy (human swayback). Mayo Clin Proc 2006;81(10):1371–84.

59. Halfdanarson TR, Kumar N, Hogan WJ, et al. Copper deficiency in celiac disease. J Clin Gastroenterol 2009;43(2):162–4.

60. Cousins RJ. Absorption, transport, and hepatic metabolism of copper and zinc: special reference to metallothionein and ceruloplasmin. Physiol Rev 1985;65(2):238–309.

61. Prodan CI, Holland NR, Wisdom PJ, et al. CNS demyelination associated with copper deficiency and hyperzincemia. Neurology 2002;59(9):1453–6.

62. Wahlin S, Harper P. The role of BMT in erythropoietic protoporphyria. Bone Marrow Transplant 2010;45(2):393–4.

63. Casas KA, Fischel-Ghodsian N. Mitochondrial myopathy and sideroblastic anemia. Am J Med Genet 2004;125A(2):201–4.

64. Fernandez-Vizarra E, Berardinelli A, Valente L, et al. Nonsense mutation in pseudouridylate synthase 1 (PUS1) in two brothers affected by myopathy, lactic acidosis and sideroblastic anemia (MLASA). J Med Genet 2007;44(3):173–80.

65. Sasarman F, Nishimura T, Thiffault I, et al. A novel mutation in YARS2 causes myopathy with lactic acidosis and sideroblastic anemia. Hum Mutat 2012; 33(8):1201–6.
66. Shahni R, Wedatilake Y, Cleary MA, et al. A distinct mitochondrial myopathy, lactic acidosis and sideroblastic anemia (MLASA) phenotype associates with YARS2 mutations. Am J Med Genet A 2013;161(9):2334–8.
67. Nakajima J, Eminoglu TF, Vatansever G, et al. A novel homozygous YARS2 mutation causes severe myopathy, lactic acidosis, and sideroblastic anemia 2. J Hum Genet 2014;59(4):229–32.
68. Ricketts CJ, Minton JA, Samuel J, et al. Thiamine-responsive megaloblastic anemia syndrome; long-term follow-up and mutation analysis of seven families. Acta Paediatr 2006;95(1):99–104.
69. Cazzola M, Barosi G, Gobbi PG, et al. Natural history of idiopathic refractory sideroblastic anemia. Blood 1988;71(2):305–12.
70. Germing U, Gattermann N, Aivado M, et al. Two types of acquired idiopathic sideroblastic anaemia (AISA): a time-tested distinction. Br J Haematol 2000; 108(4):724–8.
71. Byrd RB, Cooper T. Hereditary–iron loading anemia with secondary hemochromatosis. Ann Intern Med 1961;55:103–23.
72. Bottomley SS. Sideroblastic anemia: death from iron overload. Hosp Pract 1991; 26(Suppl 3):55–6.
73. Cotter PD, Rucknagel DI, Bishop DF. X-linked sideroblastic anemia: identification of the mutation in the erythroid-specific δ-aminolevulinate synthase gene (ALAS2) in the original family described by Cooley. Blood 1994;84(11):3915–24.
74. Aleali SH, Castro O, Spencer RP, et al. Sideroblastic anemia with splenic abscess and fatal thromboemboli after splenectomy. Ann Intern Med 1975;83(5): 661–3.
75. Byrne MT, Bergmann AK, Ruiz I, et al. Postsplenectomy thromboembolic disease. BMJ Case Rep 2010;2010. http://dx.doi.org/10.1136b/ber.12.2009.2514. pii:ber1220092514.
76. Bottomley SS. Secondary iron overload disorders. Semin Hematol 1998;35(1): 77–86.
77. Bottomley SS. Iron overload in sideroblastic and other non-thalassemic anemias. In: Barton JC, Edwards CQ, editors. Hemochromatosis, pathophysiology, diagnosis and treatment. Cambridge (United Kingdom): Cambridge University Press; 2000. p. 442–52.
78. Hathway D, Harris JW, Stenger RJ. Histopathology of the liver in pyridoxine-responsive anemia. Arch Pathol Lab Med 1967;83(2):175–9.
79. Peto TEA, Pippard MJ, Weatherall DJ. Iron overload in mild sideroblastic anaemias. Lancet 1983;1(8321):375–8.
80. Fairbanks VF, Dickson ER, Tompson ME. Hereditary sideroblastic anemia. Hosp Pract 1991;26(Suppl 3):53–5.
81. Barton JC, Lee PL. Disparate phenotype expression of ALAS2 B452H (nt 1407 G→A) in two brothers, one with severe sideroblastic anemia and iron overload, hepatic cirrhosis, and hepatocellular carcinoma. Blood Cells Mol Dis 2006; 36(3):342–6.
82. Cuijpers ML, van Spronsen DJ, Muus P, et al. Need for early recognition and therapeutic guidelines of congenital sideroblastic anaemia. Int J Hematol 2011;94(1): 97–100.
83. Pippard MJ, Weatherall DJ. Iron absorption in non-transfused iron loading anaemias: prediction of risk for iron loading and response to iron chelation treatment,

in β thalassemia intermedia and congenital sideroblastic anaemias. Haematologia (Budap) 1984;17(1):17–24.

84. Tanno T, Bhanu NV, Oneal PA, et al. High levels of GDF15 in thalassemia suppress expression of the iron regulatory protein hepcidin. Nat Med 2007;13(9): 1096–101.

85. Tanno T, Miller JL. Iron loading and overloading due to ineffective erythropoiesis. Adv Hematol 2010;2010:358283.

86. Tanno T, Noel P, Miller JL. Growth differentiation factor 15 in erythroid health and disease. Curr Opin Hematol 2010;17(3):184–90.

87. Tanno T, Porayette P, Sripichai O, et al. Identification of TWSG1 as a second novel erythroid regulator of hepcidin expression in murine and human cells. Blood 2009;114(1):181–6.

88. Kautz L, Jung G, Nemeth E, et al. The erythroid factor erythroferrone and its role in iron homeostasis [abstract]. Blood 2013;122(21):4.

89. Finch C. Regulation of iron balance in humans. Blood 1994;84(6):1697–702.

90. Malcovati L. Impact of transfusion dependency and secondary iron overload on the survival of patients with myelodysplastic syndromes. Leuk Res 2007; 31(Suppl 3):S2–6.

91. Leitch HA, Leger CS, Goodman TA, et al. Improved survival in patients with myelodysplastic syndrome receiving iron chelation therapy. Clinical Leukemia 2008; 2(3):205–11.

92. Neukirchen J, Fox F, Kundgen A, et al. Improved survival in MDS patients receiving iron chelation therapy–a matched pair analysis of 188 patients from the Dusseldorf MDS registry. Leuk Res 2012;36(8):1067–70.

93. Porter JB, Lin KH, Beris P, et al. Response of iron overload to deferasirox in rare transfusion-dependent anaemias: equivalent effects on serum ferritin and labile iron for haemolytic or production anaemias. Eur J Haematol 2011;87(4):338–48.

94. Steensma DP, Gattermann N. When is iron overload deleterious, and when and how should iron chelation therapy be administered in myelodysplastic syndromes? Best Pract Res Clin Haematol 2013;26(4):431–44.

95. Viprakasit V, Gattermann N, Lee JW, et al. Geographical variations in current clinical practice on transfusions and iron chelation therapy across various transfusion-dependent anaemias. Blood Transfus 2013;11(1):108–22.

96. Bennett JM, MDS Foundation's Working Group on Transfusional Iron Overload. Consensus statement on iron overload in myelodysplastic syndromes. Am J Hematol 2008;83(11):858–61.

97. Gattermann N. Pathophysiological and clinical aspects of iron chelation therapy in MDS. Curr Pharm Des 2012;18(22):3222–34.

98. French TJ, Jacobs P. Sideroblastic anaemia associated with iron overload treated by repeated phlebotomy. S Afr Med J 1976;50(15):594–6.

99. Badawi MA, Vickars LM, Chase JM, et al. Red blood cell transfusion independence following the initiation of iron chelation therapy in myelodysplastic syndrome. Adv Hematol 2010;2010:164045.

100. Gattermann N, Finelli C, Della Porta M, et al. Haematologic responses to deferasirox therapy in transfusion-dependent patients with myelodysplastic syndromes. Haematologica 2012;97(9):1364–71.

Anemia of Inflammation

Elizabeta Nemeth, PhD[a], Tomas Ganz, MD, PhD[a,b,*]

KEYWORDS

- Anemia of chronic disease • Hepcidin • Ferroportin • Cytokines
- Erythropoiesis-stimulating agents

KEY POINTS

- Anemia of inflammation results from hepcidin-induced hypoferremia combined with cytokine-mediated suppression of erythropoiesis and decreased lifespan of erythrocytes.
- Treatment of the cause of inflammation improves the anemia.
- Treatment with erythropoiesis-stimulating agents and/or intravenous iron is rarely necessary.

CLINICAL PRESENTATION

- Mild to moderate anemia (hemoglobin rarely <8 g/dL)
- Occurring in a setting of infection, inflammatory disease, or malignancy
- Low serum iron
- Systemic iron stores not depleted

Definitions

Anemia of inflammation (AI, formerly also called anemia of chronic disease or anemia of chronic disorders) is usually a mild to moderately severe anemia (hemoglobin rarely lower than 8 g/dL) that develops in the setting of infection, inflammatory disease, or malignancy.[1] The defining biochemical features of AI include low serum iron despite adequate systemic iron stores. The concentration of serum transferrin is also decreased during chronic inflammation but this is a lagging indicator because of the long half-life of transferrin (about 8 days) compared with iron (about 1.5 hours).[2] The erythrocytes are usually of normal size and have normal hemoglobin content but are reduced in number (normocytic, normochromic anemia). In some cases, particularly if the inflammatory disease is longstanding, the red cells are mildly decreased in size and hemoglobin content.

---

[a] Department of Medicine, David Geffen School of Medicine at UCLA, 37-055 CHS, 10833 Le Conte Avenue, Los Angeles, CA 90095, USA; [b] Department of Pathology, David Geffen School of Medicine at UCLA, 10833 Le Conte Avenue, Los Angeles, CA 90095, USA
* Corresponding author. Department of Medicine, David Geffen School of Medicine at UCLA, 37-055 CHS, 10833 Le Conte Avenue, Los Angeles, CA 90095.
E-mail address: tganz@mednet.ucla.edu

Hematol Oncol Clin N Am 28 (2014) 671–681
http://dx.doi.org/10.1016/j.hoc.2014.04.005
0889-8588/14/$ – see front matter © 2014 Elsevier Inc. All rights reserved.

Related Conditions

Anemia of critical illness presents with a similar pattern of findings but develops within days in patients who are hospitalized in intensive care units with infections, sepsis, or other inflammatory conditions.[3] Anemia of critical illness may be exacerbated by frequent diagnostic phlebotomies or increased gastrointestinal blood loss as is common in such settings. Anemia of aging[4] is a chronic anemia similar to AI but often occurring in the elderly without a specific diagnosis of a predisposing underlying disease. The prevalence of this anemia increases with age, and detailed studies often detect evidence of inflammation, including increased serum C-reactive protein or other biomarkers of inflammation. Anemia of chronic kidney disease is commonly attributed to erythropoietin deficiency but accumulating evidence favors a more complex pathogenesis with a large component of AI whose exacerbations may be manifested as "erythropoietin resistance".[5]

Diagnosis

The traditional gold standard for the diagnosis of AI was anemia with hypoferremia or with low transferrin saturation, despite the presence of Prussian blue stainable iron in bone marrow macrophages. The main confounding diagnostic entity that also presents with anemia and hypoferremia is iron deficiency anemia where there is no stainable iron in the marrow macrophages. This gold standard has been challenged not only because of the invasive nature of the marrow sampling procedure but also because of findings that bone marrow iron readings are qualitative and not always consistent between evaluators and in multiple specimens[6,7] and that iron therapy may cause marrow iron deposition in a poorly bioavailable form, which cannot be used by iron-deficient patients.[8] The marrow iron stain has largely been replaced by serum ferritin determinations. Low serum ferritin (less than 15 ng/mL for general population, with some laboratories using age and gender-specific norms) is highly specific for iron deficiency[9] (genetic deficiency of L-ferritin is an extremely rare exception[10]) and effectively rules out AI. AI is diagnosed when anemia and hypoferremia are accompanied by serum ferritin that is not low. Serum ferritin is increased by inflammation, in part reflecting direct inflammatory regulation of ferroportin synthesis[11,12] and in part because serum ferritin originates in macrophages where its synthesis is increased by iron sequestration[13] that takes place during inflammation. Iron deficiency is presumed to coexist with AI when ferritin is insufficiently elevated for the intensity of inflammation. Serum ferritin is also increased by tissue injury, especially to the liver.

Diagnostic Challenges

The determination of what constitutes "inappropriately low" ferritin may be difficult in practice because even patients with very high serum ferritin levels may respond to intravenous iron therapy by increasing hemoglobin.[14] In principle, the limitations of serum ferritin could be circumvented by assaying additional markers of iron deficiency less affected by inflammation, most prominently soluble transferrin receptor.[15–17] However, the relevant assays have not been standardized, the added value of such studies has not yet been convincingly demonstrated,[18] and none have been widely adopted. When the anemia is clinically significant and a component of iron deficiency is suspected in a patient with AI, it may be reasonable to perform a therapeutic trial of intravenous iron. Current intravenous iron preparations are quite safe, but the very rare reactions to their administration and the possibility of exacerbating an existing or occult infectious process should be included in the risk-benefit analysis.[19]

Prevalence

Detailed statistics about the prevalence of AI are not available. It is estimated that the aging of the population and the high prevalence of chronic infections and inflammatory disorders worldwide combine to make AI the second most common cause of anemia worldwide, after iron deficiency. The order may eventually reverse as iron deficiency anemia is more effectively treated or prevented by dietary iron supplementation and by public health measures that curb intestinal parasitic infections.

PATHOPHYSIOLOGY

- Mildly shortened erythrocyte survival (increased destruction)
- Hypoferremia, iron-restricted erythropoiesis from cytokine-stimulated hepcidin increase
- Suppression of erythropoiesis by direct effects of cytokines on the marrow
- Variable effects of inflammation on erythropoietin production, renal excretion of hepcidin

Overview of the Causative Factors

Despite more than 50 years of investigation, our understanding of the pathophysiology of AI is incomplete. Already the earliest studies of AI indicated that the disorder is a consequence of a mild decrease in erythrocyte survival combined with impaired production of erythrocytes.[1,20] The increased destruction of erythrocytes is predominantly attributable to macrophage activation by inflammatory cytokines but other hemolytic mechanisms may contribute in specific inflammatory diseases. The suppression of erythrocyte production has 2 major components, iron restriction and direct cytokine effects on erythropoietic progenitors. These effects combine to limit the erythropoietic response to erythropoietin, which becomes insufficient to compensate for the increased destruction of erythrocytes. In some situations, the production of erythropoietin may also be decreased, perhaps due to cytokine effects on the renal cells that produce the hormone. In severe inflammation, or when the primary pathology involves the kidneys, decreased renal excretion of hepcidin contributes to hepcidin accumulation and iron restriction.[21] The complex pathogenesis of AI is summarized in **Fig. 1** and discussed further.

Erythrocyte Destruction

Experiments with transfused erythrocytes showed that erythrocytes from AI patients and from normal controls survived longer in healthy recipients than in patients with AI.[20] The shortened survival of erythrocytes in AI has been attributed to macrophage activation by inflammatory cytokines that causes the macrophages to ingest and destroy erythrocytes prematurely. Anemia and excessive erythrophagocytosis are prominent features of macrophage activation syndromes, especially those associated with systemic juvenile rheumatoid arthritis.[22] Here, treatment targeting interleukin 1 (IL-1) or IL-6 is proving effective, suggesting an important (although possibly indirect) role of these cytokines in the pathogenesis of excessive erythrophagocytosis. In mouse models, multiple cytokines, including interferon-γ and IL-4, have been implicated in activating macrophages for erythrophagocytosis.[23,24] With the exception of fulminant hemophagocytic states, which are fortunately rare, erythrophagocytosis in AI is only mildly increased and could be readily compensated if the production of erythrocytes was not also impaired.[1,20]

Hypoferremia

A recent review of mechanisms governing iron homeostasis is provided elsewhere.[25] Briefly, plasma iron concentrations are under homeostatic control of the hepatic iron

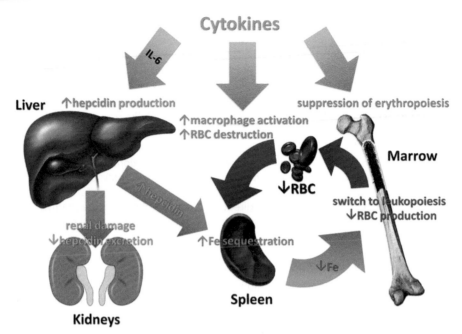

Fig. 1. The pathogenesis of AI is mediated by inflammatory cytokines and hepcidin, acting together to suppress erythropoiesis and shorten erythrocyte survival in blood. The effects of cytokines are denoted in light green, hepcidin effects in orange, and combined effects in red.

regulatory hormone hepcidin[26] and are normally maintained in the 10 to 30 μM range. Hepcidin acts by regulating the iron delivery to plasma from macrophages that recycle senescent erythrocytes, from duodenal enterocytes that absorb dietary iron, and from hepatocytes involved in iron storage. The molecular target of hepcidin is the sole known cellular iron exporter ferroportin,[27] expressed on cell membranes in tissues that deliver iron to plasma. The binding of hepcidin to ferroportin causes ferroportin endocytosis and its subsequent proteolysis in lysosomes. The loss of ferroportin from cell membranes causes a proportional reduction of iron export to plasma. The production of hepcidin by hepatocytes is in turn regulated by plasma and hepatic iron concentrations and inflammatory cytokines, chiefly IL-6.[28,29] Inflammatory stimuli administered to humans[30] or experimental animals elicit a decrease in serum iron concentration within a few hours. The response depends on inflammation-induced increase in plasma concentrations of hepcidin.[31] Increased hepcidin degrades cellular ferroportin and traps iron in macrophages, hepatocytes, and intestinal enterocytes so that less iron is delivered to plasma transferrin. The plasma iron compartment is then rapidly depleted of iron through continuing iron uptake by erythroid precursors.

Increased Hepcidin Causes an Iron-Restricted Anemia Even in the Absence of Inflammation

An experiment of nature, the syndrome of iron-refractory iron deficiency anemia (IRIDA),[32] provides an important insight into the role of hepcidin in the regulation of erythropoiesis and as a pathogenic component of AI. The otherwise healthy children with IRIDA suffer from a severely microcytic, hypochromic anemia and hypoferremia that respond poorly to treatment with oral iron and incompletely even to treatment with intravenous (IV) iron.[33,34] Guided by a mouse model of this condition,[35] the pathogenesis of IRIDA is now partially understood.[36] Most of the patients with IRIDA have homozygous or compound heterozygous mutations in the gene encoding the transmembrane serine protease TMPRSS6 (also called matriptase-2), leading to serum hepcidin levels that are high or inappropriately elevated considering that the patients are iron deficient. Hepcidin-mediated block in duodenal iron absorption is likely responsible for the ineffectiveness of oral iron therapy, and hepcidin-induced retention of iron in macrophages reduces the response to IV iron replacement therapy. Importantly, IRIDA patients continue to have microcytosis and hypochromia even after iron therapy, indicating that hemoglobin synthesis is impaired more than the production of erythrocytes. This is in contrast to AI, which is usually a normochromic normocytic anemia, indicating that in AI the impairment of hemoglobin synthesis is roughly balanced by decreased production of erythrocytes. Thus, direct suppression of erythrocyte production by inflammatory cytokines in AI may "compensate" for the effect of hypoferremia on hemoglobin synthesis, generating fewer erythrocytes but with normal size and hemoglobin content.

Suppression of Erythropoiesis by Inflammation

Inflammatory cytokines, including tumor necrosis factor (TNF) α, IL-1, and interferon-γ, have been reported to suppress erythropoiesis in vitro[37–41] as well as in mouse models.[24,42] Detailed understanding of the mechanisms involved has been hindered by the complexity of cytokine effects and the ability of each cytokine to regulate the production of many other cytokines.[41] Nevertheless, several new and promising concepts about the effects of cytokines on erythropoiesis have recently emerged. Libregts and colleagues[24] developed a mouse model where overproduction of interferon-γ leads to the development of a mild-to-moderate normocytic, normochromic anemia. The model manifests a 50% decrease in erythrocyte survival attributable to interferon-γ–mediated activation of macrophages in the splenic red pulp. The model also shows suppression of erythrocyte production affecting the erythroblast stages and the earliest erythroid-committed precursor burst-forming unit–erythrocyte but not proerythroblasts and colony-forming unit–erythrocyte (CFU-E). Importantly, myeloid CFU-granulocyte/macrophage colonies were increased. Microarray analysis of erythroblasts indicated that interferon-γ promotes the transcription of PU.1 and its target genes in an interferon regulatory factor 1–dependent manner but does not affect GATA-1 or its targets. PU.1 and GATA-1 antagonize each other's activity, so the increase in PU.1 would be expected to promote myelopoiesis at the expense of erythropoiesis. During infections with viruses or intracellular pathogens known to induce interferon-γ, this mechanism may assure sufficient production of monocytes and macrophages, at the expense of temporary impairment of erythropoiesis. Whether other inflammatory cytokines use a similar or different mechanism remains to be determined.

Hepcidin-induced Hypoferremia and Interferon-γ Synergize to Suppress Erythropoiesis

Richardson and colleagues[43] examined how inflammatory cytokines and hypoferremia interact to affect erythropoiesis during AI. Using in vitro culture of human CD34+ primary progenitors, they documented that hypoferremia (transferrin saturation $\leq 15\%$) potentiates the suppressive effects of TNF-α and interferon-γ on erythropoiesis. Surprisingly, erythropoietic suppression could be reversed by the addition of the Krebs cycle intermediate isocitrate, a product of the enzyme aconitase, which also functions as a cellular iron sensor. Isocitrate injections also reversed AI in a rat model of autoimmune arthritis induced by injection of streptococcal peptidoglycan-polysaccharide. The authors present evidence that hypoferremia activates PU.1 via a protein kinase C pathway, synergizing with the effect of interferon-γ. Isocitrate, acting on aconitase, reverses the effect of hypoferremia on PU.1 and relieves the suppression of erythropoiesis. It remains to be seen if these effects are important in other animal models and in human subjects.

Animal Models of AI Show Partial Dependence on Hepcidin

A new mouse model of AI was generated by a single intraperitoneal injection of heat-killed *Brucella abortus*.[44] Like human AI, this model showed multifactorial pathogenesis including iron restriction from increased hepcidin, transient suppression of erythropoiesis, and shortened erythrocyte lifespan. Mice developed severe anemia with mild microcytosis and mild hypochromia, a hemoglobin nadir at 14 days and partial recovery by 28 days.[45,46] After an early increase in inflammatory markers and hepcidin, the mice manifested hypoferremia despite iron accumulation in the liver. Erythropoiesis was suppressed between days 1 and 7, and erythrocyte destruction was increased as evidenced by shortened red blood cell lifespan and rare schistocytes on blood smears. Erythropoietic recovery began after 14 days but was iron-restricted, as documented by increased erythrocyte zinc protoporphyrin. In mice with ablated hepcidin-1 gene, anemia was milder, not iron-restricted, and with faster recovery, supporting the role of hepcidin in the development of AI.

In the same mouse model of AI, the therapeutic administration of antihepcidin monoclonal antibodies decreased the severity of anemia.[44,47] Moreover, resistance to exogenous erythropoietin doses observed in this model was relieved by coadministration of the antibodies with erythropoietin. In the rat model of autoimmune arthritis induced by injection of streptococcal peptidoglycan-polysaccharide, suppressing hepcidin production by administration of the dorsomorphin derivative LDN-193189 or soluble hemojuvelin-Fc fusion protein, 2 agents that interfere with bone morphogenetic protein receptor signaling, also ameliorated anemia.[48]

TREATMENT OF AI

- Treat the underlying disease
- Treat anemia specifically only if severe or limits activities of daily living
- Erythrocyte transfusion for acute symptoms
- Erythropoiesis-stimulating agents (ESAs) with or without IV iron (off-label treatment)
- Experimental therapies under development include new ESAs, anticytokine drugs, and agents targeting the hepcidin-ferroportin pathway

Current Therapy

AI is a secondary manifestation of inflammatory disorders, and treating the underlying disease will correct the anemia. Such treatment is not always possible. Direct treatment of anemia should be considered only if it is impairing the patient's performance, quality of life, or recovery from underlying illness. Inflammatory diseases sufficiently severe to cause AI may also cause fatigue or malaise through cytokine-dependent mechanisms, so these symptoms need not be caused by anemia. Potential therapies for AI include erythrocyte transfusions usually reserved for severe and acutely symptomatic anemia, and ESAs (erythropoietin and its derivatives, mimics or inducers, as they become available) with or without intravenous iron supplementation. AI is not a specifically approved indication for the use of ESAs but should be considered as an

Table 1
Experimental therapeutics for the treatment of AI (not including ESAs)

Agent or Activity	Target	Chemistry	Development Status	Key Published Results
Tocilizumab	IL-6 receptor	Humanized monoclonal antibody	Approved to treat rheumatoid arthritis and juvenile rheumatoid arthritis (Genentech, Roche, Chugai)	Tocilizumab rapidly reduced hepcidin levels and improved anemia in patients with Castleman syndrome[55] or rheumatoid arthritis[56,57]
Siltuximab	IL-6	Chimeric mouse-human monoclonal antibody	Submitted for FDA approval for multifocal Castleman disease (Janssen)	Siltuximab lowered hepcidin and improved anemia in patients with renal cell carcinoma[58]
Hepcidin binders	Hepcidin peptide	Monoclonal antibody	Preclinical to phase 1 (Lilly)	
		Anticalins	Preclinical (Pieris)	PRS-080 increased serum iron in monkeys[59]
		Spiegelmers	Phase 2[a] (Noxxon)	NOX-H94 alleviated IL-6-induced anemia in a primate model[60]
Inhibitors of hepcidin production	Inhibit signaling by bone morphogenetic protein receptor type I	The kinase site of bone morphogenetic receptor I	Preclinical	LDN-193189 improved anemia in the mouse model of turpentine-induced AI[61]
	Neutralize bone morphogenetic proteins	Soluble hemojuvelin-Fc fusion protein	Phase 2a[a] (FerruMax)	Hemojuvelin-Fc fusion protein alleviated anemia in a rat model of arthritis[48] elicited by Group A streptococcal peptidoglycan-polysaccharide
		Heparin derivatives	Preclinical	Heparin reduced hepcidin expression[62] in mice and serum hepcidin concentrations in patients[62]
	Inactivate hepcidin mRNA	Antisense oligonucleotides (ASO)	Preclinical (Xenon/ISIS)	Antimouse hepcidin ASO improved anemia in a turpentine model of AI in mice[63]
	Inactivate transferrin receptor 2 mRNA	siRNA oligonucleotides	Preclinical (Alnylam)	Anti-TfR2 siRNA alleviated AI in rodent models[64]
Ferroportin blockers	Hepcidin binding site on ferroportin	Monoclonal antibody	Phase 1[a] (Lilly)	

Abbreviations: FDA, Food and Drug Administration; mRNA, messenger RNA; siRNA, small interfering RNA.
[a] Clinicaltrials.gov.

alternative to chronic erythrocyte transfusion. The use of ESAs in AI is based on a small number of anecdotal reports[49–53] that reported improvement of anemia, and similarities between AI and anemia of chronic kidney disease (CKD), the main indication for ESAs. In CKD, IV iron supplementation potentiates the effect of erythropoietin and its derivatives,[54] and it has been reported that IV iron may have a similar activity in AI.[53]

Experimental Therapy

Experimental treatments of AI target cytokines or the hepcidin-ferroportin axis and its various regulators (**Table 1**). Most of these agents have proved effective in animal models and several are undergoing human trials. Anti-IL-6 agents and other anticytokine drugs that indirectly lower IL-6 levels are already approved for the treatment of severe inflammatory diseases. Some of these agents may prove to be very effective for the treatment of AI in other settings, reflecting the important role of IL-6 in its pathogenesis. Because AI affects symptoms and quality of life but has not been demonstrated to affect survival from the underlying disease, drugs specifically targeted for AI must not only demonstrate efficacy but also be well-tolerated and free of serious side effects.

REFERENCES

1. Cartwright GE, Lee GR. The anaemia of chronic disorders. Br J Haematol 1971; 21(2):147–52.
2. Katz JH. Iron and protein kinetics studied by means of doubly labeled human crystalline transferrin. J Clin Invest 1961;40:2143–52.
3. Corwin HL, Krantz SB. Anemia of the critically ill: "acute" anemia of chronic disease. Crit Care Med 2000;28(8):3098–9.
4. Beghe C, Wilson A, Ershler WB. Prevalence and outcomes of anemia in geriatrics: a systematic review of the literature. Am J Med 2004;116(7 Suppl 1):3–10.
5. Elliott J, Mishler D, Agarwal R. Hyporesponsiveness to erythropoietin: causes and management. Adv Chronic Kidney Dis 2009;16(2):94–100.
6. Barron BA, Hoyer JD, Tefferi A. A bone marrow report of absent stainable iron is not diagnostic of iron deficiency. Ann Hematol 2001;80(3):166–9.
7. Krause JR, Brubaker D, Kaplan S. Comparison of stainable iron in aspirated and needle-biopsy specimens of bone marrow. Am J Clin Pathol 1979;72(1):68–70.
8. Thomason RW, Lavelle J, Nelson D, et al. Parenteral iron therapy is associated with a characteristic pattern of iron staining on bone marrow aspirate smears. Am J Clin Pathol 2007;128(4):590–3.
9. Ferraro S, Mozzi R, Panteghini M. Revaluating serum ferritin as a marker of body iron stores in the traceability era. Clin Chem Lab Med 2012;50(11):1911–6.
10. Cozzi A, Santambrogio P, Privitera D, et al. Human L-ferritin deficiency is characterized by idiopathic generalized seizures and atypical restless leg syndrome. J Exp Med 2013;210(9):1779–91.
11. Tran TN, Eubanks SK, Schaffer KJ, et al. Secretion of ferritin by rat hepatoma cells and its regulation by inflammatory cytokines and iron. Blood 1997; 90(12):4979–86.
12. Thomson AM, Cahill CM, Cho HH, et al. The Acute Box cis-Element in Human Heavy Ferritin mRNA 5'-Untranslated Region Is a Unique Translation Enhancer That Binds Poly(C)-binding Proteins. J Biol Chem 2005;280(34):30032–45.
13. Cohen LA, Gutierrez L, Weiss A, et al. Serum ferritin is derived primarily from macrophages through a nonclassical secretory pathway. Blood 2010;116(9): 1574–84.

14. Cazzola M, Ponchio L, de Benedetti F, et al. Defective iron supply for eryth-ropoiesis and adequate endogenous erythropoietin production in the anemia associated with systemic-onset juvenile chronic arthritis. Blood 1996;87(11): 4824–30.
15. Cook JD, Flowers CH, Skikne BS. The quantitative assessment of body iron. Blood 2003;101(9):3359–63.
16. Pettersson T, Kivivuori SM, Siimes MA. Is serum transferrin receptor useful for detecting iron-deficiency in anaemic patients with chronic inflammatory dis-eases? Br J Rheumatol 1994;33(8):740–4.
17. Skikne BS, Flowers CH, Cook JD. Serum transferrin receptor: a quantitative measure of tissue iron deficiency. Blood 1990;75(9):1870–6.
18. Infusino I, Braga F, Dolci A, et al. Soluble transferrin receptor (sTfR) and sTfR/log ferritin index for the diagnosis of iron-deficiency anemia a meta-analysis. Am J Clin Pathol 2012;138(5):642–9.
19. Litton E, Xiao J, Ho KM. Safety and efficacy of intravenous iron therapy in reducing requirement for allogeneic blood transfusion: systematic review and meta-analysis of randomised clinical trials. BMJ 2013;347:f4822.
20. Freireich EJ, Ross JF, Bayles TB, et al. Radioactive iron metabolism and eryth-rocyte survival studies of the mechanism of the anemia associated with rheuma-toid arthritis. J Clin Invest 1957;36(7):1043–58.
21. Troutt JS, Butterfield AM, Konrad RJ. Hepcidin-25 concentrations are markedly increased in patients with chronic kidney disease and are inversely correlated with estimated glomerular filtration rates. J Clin Lab Anal 2013;27(6):504–10.
22. Correll CK, Binstadt BA. Advances in the pathogenesis and treatment of sys-temic juvenile idiopathic arthritis. Pediatr Res 2014;75(1–2):176–83.
23. Milner JD, Orekov T, Ward JM, et al. Sustained IL-4 exposure leads to a novel pathway for hemophagocytosis, inflammation, and tissue macrophage accumu-lation. Blood 2010;116(14):2476–83.
24. Libregts SF, Gutierrez L, de Bruin AM, et al. Chronic IFN-gamma production in mice induces anemia by reducing erythrocyte life span and inhibiting erythro-poiesis through an IRF-1/PU.1 axis. Blood 2011;118(9):2578–88.
25. Ganz T. Systemic iron homeostasis. Physiol Rev 2013;93(4):1721–41.
26. Ganz T, Nemeth E. Hepcidin and iron homeostasis. Biochim Biophys Acta 2012; 1823(9):1434–43.
27. Nemeth E, Tuttle MS, Powelson J, et al. Hepcidin regulates cellular iron efflux by binding to ferroportin and inducing its internalization. Science 2004;306(5704): 2090–3.
28. Nemeth E, Rivera S, Gabayan V, et al. IL-6 mediates hypoferremia of inflamma-tion by inducing the synthesis of the iron regulatory hormone hepcidin. J Clin Invest 2004;113(9):1271–6.
29. Rodriguez R, Jung CL, Gabayan V, et al. Hepcidin induction by pathogens and pathogen-derived molecules is strongly dependent on interleukin-6. Infect Im-mun 2014;82(2):745–52.
30. Kemna E, Pickkers P, Nemeth E, et al. Time-course analysis of hepcidin, serum iron, and plasma cytokine levels in humans injected with LPS. Blood 2005; 106(5):1864–6.
31. Nicolas G, Chauvet C, Viatte L, et al. The gene encoding the iron regulatory pep-tide hepcidin is regulated by anemia, hypoxia, and inflammation. J Clin Invest 2002;110(7):1037–44.
32. Finberg KE, Heeney MM, Campagna DR, et al. Mutations in TMPRSS6 cause iron-refractory iron deficiency anemia (IRIDA). Nat Genet 2008;40(5):569–71.

33. Finberg KE. Iron-refractory iron deficiency anemia. Semin Hematol 2009;46(4): 378–86.
34. Camaschella C, Poggiali E. Inherited disorders of iron metabolism. Curr Opin Pediatr 2011;23(1):14–20.
35. Du X, She E, Gelbart T, et al. The serine protease TMPRSS6 is required to sense iron deficiency. Science 2008;320(5879):1088–92.
36. Silvestri L, Pagani A, Nai A, et al. The serine protease matriptase-2 (TMPRSS6) inhibits hepcidin activation by cleaving membrane hemojuvelin. Cell Metab 2008;8(6):502–11.
37. Means RT Jr, Krantz SB. Inhibition of human erythroid colony-forming units by tumor necrosis factor requires beta interferon. J Clin Invest 1993;91(2):416–9.
38. Means RT Jr, Dessypris EN, Krantz SB. Inhibition of human erythroid colony-forming units by interleukin-1 is mediated by gamma interferon. J Cell Physiol 1992;150(1):59–64.
39. Means RT Jr, Krantz SB. Inhibition of human erythroid colony-forming units by gamma interferon can be corrected by recombinant human erythropoietin. Blood 1991;78(10):2564–7.
40. Broxmeyer HE, Williams DE, Lu L, et al. The suppressive influences of human tumor necrosis factors on bone marrow hematopoietic progenitor cells from normal donors and patients with leukemia: synergism of tumor necrosis factor and interferon-gamma. J Immunol 1986;136(12):4487–95.
41. Felli N, Pedini F, Zeuner A, et al. Multiple members of the TNF superfamily contribute to IFN-γmediated inhibition of erythropoiesis. J Immunol 2005; 175(3):1464–72.
42. Johnson RA, Waddelow TA, Caro J, et al. Chronic exposure to tumor necrosis factor in vivo preferentially inhibits erythropoiesis in nude mice. Blood 1989; 74(1):130–8.
43. Richardson CL, Delehanty LL, Bullock GC, et al. Isocitrate ameliorates anemia by suppressing the erythroid iron restriction response. J Clin Invest 2013; 123(8):3614–23.
44. Sasu BJ, Cooke KS, Arvedson TL, et al. Antihepcidin antibody treatment modulates iron metabolism and is effective in a mouse model of inflammation-induced anemia. Blood 2010;115(17):3616–24.
45. Gardenghi S, Renaud TM, Meloni A, et al. Distinct roles for hepcidin and interleukin-6 in the recovery from anemia in mice injected with heat-killed Brucella abortus. Blood 2014;123(8):1137–45.
46. Kim A, Fung E, Parikh SG, et al. A mouse model of anemia of inflammation: complex pathogenesis with partial dependence on hepcidin. Blood 2014;123(8):1129–36.
47. Cooke KS, Hinkle B, Salimi-Moosavi H, et al. A fully human anti-hepcidin antibody modulates iron metabolism in both mice and nonhuman primates. Blood 2013;122(17):3054–61.
48. Theurl I, Schroll A, Sonnweber T, et al. Pharmacologic inhibition of hepcidin expression reverses anemia of chronic inflammation in rats. Blood 2011; 118(18):4977–84.
49. Kato Y, Takagi C, Tanaka J, et al. Effect of daily subcutaneous administration of recombinant erythropoietin on chronic anemia in rheumatoid arthritis. Intern Med 1994;33(4):193–7.
50. Peeters HR, Jongen-Lavrencic M, Bakker CH, et al. Recombinant human erythropoietin improves health-related quality of life in patients with rheumatoid arthritis and anaemia of chronic disease; utility measures correlate strongly with disease activity measures. Rheumatol Int 1999;18(5–6):201–6.

51. Peeters HR, Jongen-Lavrencic M, Vreugdenhil G, et al. Effect of recombinant human erythropoietin on anaemia and disease activity in patients with rheumatoid arthritis and anaemia of chronic disease: a randomised placebo controlled double blind 52 weeks clinical trial. Ann Rheum Dis 1996;55(10):739–44.
52. Pettersson T, Rosenlof K, Friman C, et al. Successful treatment of the anemia of rheumatoid arthritis with subcutaneously administered recombinant human erythropoietin. Slower response in patients with more severe inflammation. Scand J Rheumatol 1993;22(4):188–93.
53. Arndt U, Kaltwasser JP, Gottschalk R, et al. Correction of iron-deficient erythropoiesis in the treatment of anemia of chronic disease with recombinant human erythropoietin. Ann Hematol 2005;84(3):159–66.
54. Singh A. Hemoglobin control, ESA resistance, and regular low-dose IV iron therapy: a review of the evidence. Semin Dial 2009;22(1):64–9.
55. Song SN, Tomosugi N, Kawabata H, et al. Down-regulation of hepcidin resulting from long-term treatment with an anti-IL-6 receptor antibody (tocilizumab) improves anemia of inflammation in multicentric Castleman disease. Blood 2010; 116(18):3627–34.
56. Song SN, Iwahashi M, Tomosugi N, et al. Comparative evaluation of the effects of treatment with tocilizumab and TNF-alpha inhibitors on serum hepcidin, anemia response and disease activity in rheumatoid arthritis patients. Arthritis Res Ther 2013;15(5):R141.
57. Isaacs JD, Harari O, Kobold U, et al. Effect of tocilizumab on haematological markers implicates interleukin-6 signalling in the anaemia of rheumatoid arthritis. Arthritis Res Ther 2013;15(6):R204.
58. Schipperus M, Rijnbeek B, Reddy M, et al. CNTO328 (Anti-IL-6 mAb) treatment is associated with an increase in hemoglobin (Hb) and decrease in hepcidin levels in renal cell carcinoma (RCC) [abstract]. Blood 2009;22(114):4045.
59. Hohlbaum A, Gille H, Christian J, et al. Iron mobilization and pharmacodynic marker measurements in non-human primates following administration of PRS-080, a novel and highly specific anti-hepcidin therapeutic [abstract]. Am J Hematol 2013;88(5):E41.
60. Schwoebel F, van Eijk LT, Zboralski D, et al. The effects of the anti-hepcidin Spiegelmer NOX-H94 on inflammation-induced anemia in cynomolgus monkeys. Blood 2013;121(12):2311–5.
61. Steinbicker AU, Sachidanandan C, Vonner AJ, et al. Inhibition of bone morphogenetic protein signaling attenuates anemia associated with inflammation. Blood 2011;117(18):4915–23.
62. Poli M, Girelli D, Campostrini N, et al. Heparin: a potent inhibitor of hepcidin expression in vitro and in vivo. Blood 2011;117(3):997–1004.
63. Crosby JR, Gaarde WA, Egerston J, et al. Targeting hepcidin with antisense oligonucletides improves anemia endpoints in mice. Blood 2006;108(11 Pt 1): 83A–4A.
64. Akinc A, Chan-Daniels A, Sehgal A, et al. Targeting the Hepcidin Pathway with RNAi Therapeutics for the Treatment of Anemia. Blood 2011;118(21):315.

The Pathophysiology of Transfusional Iron Overload

 CrossMark

John B. Porter, MD*, Maciej Garbowski, MD

KEYWORDS

- Iron overload • Pathophysiology • Mechanism • Thalassemia • Sickle cell disease
- Blood transfusion • NTBI • Extra-hepatic iron distribution

KEY POINTS

- The pathophysiologic consequences of transfusional iron overload (TIO) are best under-stood in thalassemia major (TM) and broadly reflect the distribution of excess storage iron to heart, endocrine tissues, and liver.
- The pattern of excess iron distribution reflects the pattern of nontransferrin-bound iron (NTBI) uptake to these tissues.
- Storage iron does not directly damage cells but its intracellular turnover contributes to labile intracellular iron pools that generate harmful free radicals.
- TIO also increases the risk of infection due to increased availability of labile iron to microorganisms.
- In other conditions such as sickle cell disease, Diamond-Blackfan anemia, and myelodys-plastic syndrome, the propensity to the extrahepatic iron distribution and its conse-quences vary compared with TM.
- The mechanisms underlining this variability may reflect differences in the transfusional iron loading rates, age of commencing transfusion, as well as differences between transferrin iron utilization and NTBI generation.

IRON HOMEOSTATIC MECHANISMS

Iron homeostatic mechanisms are key to the pathophysiology of transfusional iron overload (TIO). In humans, these mechanisms are best adapted to increasing iron acquisition in conditions of iron deficiency or anemia, or to limiting iron distribution from the macrophage system during inflammation. They are not well adapted, how-ever, to controlling the distribution of TIO or to eliminating excess iron. This is in

Dr Porter is supported by NIHR University College London Hospitals Biomedical Research Centre (BRC).
Department of Haematology, University College London, 72 Huntley Street, London WC1E 6BT, UK
* Corresponding author.
E-mail address: j.porter@ucl.ac.uk

Hematol Oncol Clin N Am 28 (2014) 683–701
http://dx.doi.org/10.1016/j.hoc.2014.04.003
0889-8588/14/$ – see front matter © 2014 Elsevier Inc. All rights reserved.
hemonc.theclinics.com

marked contrast to rodents, where most studies on iron overload and iron metabolism have been performed and where iron overload is eliminated efficiently by the biliary route. Iron homeostasis is adapted to supplying only that which is essential for the functioning of proteins involved in oxygen transport, oxidative energy production, mitochondrial respiration, and DNA synthesis, while minimizing the potential for iron toxicity from its redox cycling. These homeostatic mechanisms work at 2 levels: firstly at the level of the whole body through interactions of plasma hepcidin with membrane ferroportin and secondly at a cellular level through interaction of iron responsive element (IRE)-binding proteins (IRPs) with IREs present on mRNAs of key iron metabolism–related proteins.

Body Iron Homeostasis

A healthy human contains 40 to 50 mg/kg of iron, mainly as hemoglobin (30 mg/kg). About 4 mg/kg is present in muscle myoglobin, with 2 mg/kg in cells as iron-containing enzymes. Storage iron, present as ferritin and its compact, partially degraded form hemosiderin, ranges from 0 to 2000 mg[1]; this is mainly present in liver, spleen, and bone marrow (BM) macrophages, formerly referred to as the reticuloendothelial system (RES), and in hepatocytes.[2] Liver iron concentration (LIC) rarely exceeds 1.8 mg/g dry weight (dw) in healthy individuals in the absence of liver disease, hemochromatosis genes, inappropriate dietary supplementation, or blood transfusion.

A healthy individual absorbs only about 10% of dietary iron or about 1 to 2 mg/d, usually balanced by iron loss from skin, gut, menstruation, or pregnancy. Anemia, hypoxia, ineffective erythropoiesis (IE), and the presence of variant HFE genes increase iron absorption, the common factor being low, or inappropriately low, plasma hepcidin levels.[3] The latter permits higher enterocyte ferroportin expression, allowing Fe(II) flux and hence increasing dietary iron absorption. Iron absorption is also increased through hypoxia-inducible factor 1–mediated signaling, by duodenal upregulation of DcytB and DMT1 expression.[4] Thus, in principle, any anemia will tend to increase the efficiency of iron absorption. Most body iron turnover, however, is not directed through iron absorption, but through plasma transferrin, which, although binding only 1 to 2 mg of iron at any moment, in a healthy adult delivers about 20 to 30 mg/d *via* transferrin receptors on the erythron for hemoglobin synthesis.

Hepcidin regulation is important both to iron absorption from diet and to iron egress from erythrophagocytic macrophages. Hepcidin controls iron egress from both macrophages and enterocytes by binding to and degrading ferroportin, through which Fe(II) exits these cells.[5,6] Hepatic hepcidin synthesis is controlled by at least 3 distinct regulatory mechanisms responsive to levels of iron, erythropoiesis, or inflammation.

- Extracellular iron sensing involves the binding of diferric transferrin to transferrin receptor 1 (TfR1), initiating the translocation of HFE from TfR1 to TfR2 and its subsequent signaling via ERK1/ERK2 and p38 MAP kinase to induce hepcidin expression. Storage iron sensing is affected by BMP6 signaling via BMP receptor (and SMADs pathway) whose sensitivity is markedly increased by its interaction with hemojuvelin, HFE, and TfR2 in holotransferrin-dependent manner, thus enhancing hepcidin transcription.[7,8]
- Erythropoiesis sensing involves BM-derived factors that suppress hepcidin synthesis; conditions with high levels of IE will have high levels of these factors, the nature of which has been debated. These include GDF15[9]; twisted gastrulation factor-1[10]; and most recently erythoferrone,[11] which has been identified as a key factor in mice, although its relevance in humans has yet to be demonstrated. Another separate erythropoiesis sensing mechanism likely involves desaturation

of transferrin by the erythron as disruption of transferrin iron uptake into erythron in *hbd* mouse increases hepcidin level despite ongoing anemia,[8,12] presumably overriding the erythropoietic depressors of hepcidin (or demonstrating that depressors have an effect only with concomitant transferrin desaturation).

- Inflammation sensing mediated through IL-6/STATs pathway and other cytokines upregulates hepcidin synthesis,[13] being the key mechanism in hypoferremia of acute inflammation through the action of ferroportin degradation in macrophages.[5]

Erythropoietic drive overrides both iron sensing[14–16] and inflammation sensing mechanisms,[17] but the extent to which these potentially opposing regulators of hepcidin synthesis play out in the context of iron metabolism in TIO is difficult to predict from murine studies alone and require careful clinical observations. These are discussed later under the clinical condition in question.

Cellular Iron Homeostasis

Intracellular iron homeostasis is controlled not only by the synthesis of ferritin but also by the regulation of iron uptake through regulation of membrane transferrin receptors (TfR). Both of these are regulated by IREs, stem-loop structures present in untranslated regions (UTR) of mRNA, for example, in the 5′UTR of H-ferritin or the 3′UTR of TfR mRNA, respectively. Both of these are sensitive to the magnitude of labile intracellular iron pools (LIP) through interaction with cellular IRPs; the conformation of IRPs and their binding to IREs are sensitive to LIP concentrations.[18] IRE binding of both IRP1 and IRP2 increases in iron-deficient conditions, but both are rapidly degraded by iron and heme. IRP2 has predominant control overall,[19] whereas IRP1 can switch from aconitase activity form in iron repletion (dependent on iron-sulphur cluster assembly, 4Fe-4S) to IRE-binding form in iron deficiency (losing iron: 3Fe-4S).[20] Therefore, both their cellular level and the position of IRE on mRNA regulate in concert the onset and degree of translation events (5′UTR governing access to matrices, 3′UTR governing stability of matrices by regulating the binding of nucleases). High levels of LIP thus increase ferritin synthesis while decreasing the membrane expression of TfR1. However, in the erythron such feedback is absent; instead *transcriptional* control permits high TfR despite high cellular iron or heme, consistent with hemoglobin synthesis requirements. Most ferroportin transcripts also contain IRE at 5′UTR, and therefore the amount of mRNA is increased in iron overload. However, the effective regulation of ferroportin happens post-translationally through hepcidin-dependent down-regulation[6] or lack of Fe(II) acceptor.[21]

The availability of iron for the synthesis of iron-containing molecules at a cellular level is directed through a transient low molecular weight iron pool, LIP, which in turn determines the levels and action of IRPs. Although LIP iron has been proposed to be coordinated mainly by glutathione from a thermodynamic perspective,[22] its exact nature still remains unclear, but it can potentially redox cycle between Fe(II) and Fe(III) with consequent generation of harmful free radicals. To minimize these risks, elegant homeostatic mechanisms carefully coordinate the distribution of body iron so as to provide iron pools for efficient synthesis of these proteins, while minimizing iron-mediated free radical generation.

IMPACT OF BLOOD TRANSFUSION ON IRON BALANCE

The rates and nature of blood transfusion regimens affect iron accumulation and its distribution in the body. This is key to the pathophysiology of iron overload and varies with the underlying clinical condition.

Thalassemia Major

In thalassemia major (TM), blood transfusion typically begins in the first year of life. Current transfusion recommendations in TM aim to keep the pretransfusion hemoglobin level at approximately 9.5 g/dL and to maintain an average hemoglobin of 12 g/dL,[23] which usually amounts to an iron load rate (ILR) of 0.3 to 0.5 mg/kg/d.[23] This regimen has been arrived at so as to balance the beneficial effects of suppression of IE and dietary iron absorption with the iron accumulated from transfusion. The transfusional suppression of the endogenous BM activity can be assessed by monitoring circulating transferrin receptors, which show more suppression when the pretransfusion hemoglobin level exceeds 10 g/dL.[24] Maintenance of a mean pretransfusion hemoglobin level of 9.4 g/dL versus 11.3 g/dL decreased net blood consumption and was associated with improved control of iron overload in Italian patients.[25] This optimal balance may not be universal and may depend on the severity of thalassemia genotype. In the prechelation era, LICs of 40 mg/g dw were typically seen by 10 years of age.[26] Failure to control these levels risks extrahepatic spread of iron (see later discussion).

Sickle Cell Disease

The age of commencing blood transfusion, transfusional ILR, and the nature of the transfusion regimen itself, all affect the rate and extent of iron overload in sickle cell disease (SCD) and often differ considerably from TM. Net iron accumulation from transfusion in SCD is slower than TM, firstly because of differences in transfusion practice between these conditions and secondly because SCD patients tend to be in negative iron balance in the absence of transfusion. In SCD, there is considerable intravascular hemolysis leading to iron loss via urine[27–29] (as in PNH) and possibly bile.[30] Urinary iron loss in SCD may reach as much as 15 mg/d (~0.2 mg/kg/d, ie, comparable to average SCD transfusional ILR).[28] Furthermore, the marrow is less expanded in SCD than in TM or NTDT, leading to less hepcidin suppression and less tendency for increased iron absorption.[31] Under conditions of hypertransfusion, where synthesis of sickle hemoglobin (HbS) is suppressed, or under vigorous chronic automated exchange procedures, where the percentage of HbS is maintained at low levels, intravascular hemolysis will also be suppressed and thus the tendency to lose iron through this mechanism will be diminished.

Historically, blood transfusions were typically sporadic and given by simple transfusion or by some form of partial exchange procedure in response to acute episodes, which over a lifetime would lead to significant iron overload. Transfusion has been increasingly given to prevent primary and secondary stroke.[32] This approach, together with a wider use of transfusion to prevent or treat other complications, such as chest syndrome, or in preparation for major surgery, puts an increasing proportion of patients at risk of TIO. In a large multicenter international study, where most patients received simple (60%) or exchange transfusions (20%), the mean ILR was 0.22 mg/kg/d,[33] notably lower than in TM. Manual exchange procedures, where about one-third of the blood volume is exchanged, lead to ILR of about 40% of simple transfusions, as estimated from ferritin increments.[34] With automated erythrocytapheresis, ILR was only 0.053 mg/kg/d with a target pretransfusion HbS less than 50%[35] compared with 0.39 mg/kg/d for simple transfusion with a target HbS less than 30% and 0.29 mg/kg/d with a target HbS less than 50%.

Other Conditions

In other forms of TIO, the rates of ILR again vary considerably; for example, a mean of 0.4 mg/kg/d was found in transfusion-dependent Diamond-Blackfan anemia (DBA) patients with 0.28 mg/kg/d in myelodysplastic syndrome (MDS) patients in the same study.[36] Patients who receive repeated myeloablative chemotherapy cycles for leukemias or lymphomas can accumulate more than 100 units of transfused blood or 20 g of excess body iron that will eventually require removal if long-term iron toxicity is to be avoided.

MECHANISMS OF IRON TOXICITY IN TRANSFUSIONAL OVERLOAD

The pathophysiologic consequences of TIO, which are broadly observed in tissues in which storage iron accumulates at the highest concentrations, are summarized in **Fig. 1**. Ferritin within cells is degraded in lysosomes or proteasomes, the iron is released into LIP, and this iron is reincorporated into new ferritin synthesis or made available for synthesis of essential iron-containing proteins.[20] Once the LIP reaches a critical concentration,[40] the iron can redox cycle between ferric Fe(III) and ferrous Fe(II) forms through the donation or acceptance of an electron and enhance the generation of reactive oxygen species (ROS), with a cascade of consequences (see **Fig. 1**). Both the concentration of LIP as well as the capacity of cells to accommodate increased levels of iron are likely to vary between cell type, and the exact nature and redox state of LIP remain unresolved. For example, in the human K562 cell line LIP concentrations of 0.24 to 0.4 μM have been estimated using the fluorochrome calcein as a probe.[41] However, using electron paramagnetic resonance (EPR) spectroscopy,

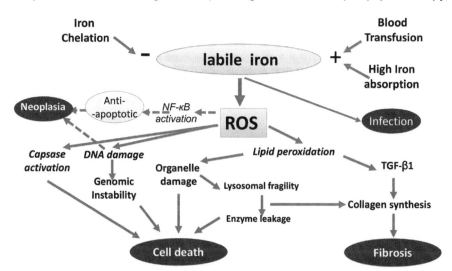

Fig. 1. Pathologic mechanisms and consequences of iron overload. In iron overload resulting from repeated blood transfusions or long-term increased iron absorption, iron that is not liganded to naturally occurring molecules, such as transferrin or ferritin or to therapeutic iron chelators, generates a variety of ROS, most notably hydroxyl radicals. This occurs in cells where storage iron is accumulated (especially liver, endocrine tissues, and myocardium) thereby increasing levels of both storage and labile cellular iron. ROS increase lipid peroxidation and organelle damage, leading to cell death and fibrogenesis mediated by transforming growth factor (TGF) β1.[37] ROS also damage DNA, risking genomic instability, mutagenesis, and cell death or neoplasia. ROS directly activates caspases thereby accelerating apoptotic death.[38] Paradoxically, ROS may also have antiapoptotic effects by activating NF-kB (*dashed lines*),[39] which may contribute to MDS transformation and to iron-mediated neoplasia such as hepatoma. (*Adapted from* Porter JB. Pathophysiology of iron overhead. Hematol Oncol Clin North Am 2005;19(Suppl 1):7–12.)

which detects Fe(III) and requires no manipulation of cells, an intracellular EPR-detectable high-spin ferric iron signal was found at approximately 3.2 μM.[42,43] More recently, increased levels of LIP have been linked to increased ROS production and potentially oncogenic effects.[44] Ferritin acts as a sink for LIP by decreasing its magnitude and its potential toxicity. For example, murine erythroleukemia cells overexpressing H-ferritin displayed lower levels of LIP and ROS.[45]

Not all ROS are necessarily toxic to cells however. Large quantities of superoxide are produced naturally by respiration (about 30 g/d of superoxide) but their toxic potential is controlled by their conversion to water by superoxide dismutase and glutathione peroxidase. It is the favorable redox potential of the Fe(II)/Fe(III) couple (between +0.35 and −0.5 V) that allows it to redox cycle and thus catalyze the interaction of superoxide with hydrogen peroxide (H_2O_2) through the Haber-Weiss reaction, generating highly reactive hydroxyl free radicals.[46] The hydroxyl radical has a great affinity for electrons, will oxidize all substances within its immediate vicinity (diffusion radius of 2.3 nm),[46] and has been shown to promote lipid peroxidation,[47,48] with damage to organelles such as lysosomes[49] and mitochondria.[50,51] The interaction of the hydroxyl radical with lipid proceeds through the initial abstraction of a hydrogen atom (to yield a water molecule); molecular rearrangement of the lipid with peroxidation; and the formation of a peroxyl radical, which is able to propagate further lipid peroxidation in a chain reaction. The end result is decomposition of lipid molecules with concomitant effects on the integrity of organelles. Although organelle damage may lead directly to apoptotic cell death,[52,53] this may also encourage fibrogenesis as iron-induced aldehyde lipid peroxidation products such as MDA[54] and 4-HNE[55] promote collagen gene expression. Fibrogenesis is also associated with autocrine production of TGFβ-1 in stellate cells (see **Fig. 1**).[56] ROS also damage DNA, risking genomic instability, mutagenesis, and cell death or neoplasia. ROS also directly activate caspases, thereby accelerating apoptosis,[38] but, paradoxically, may also have antiapoptotic effects by activating NF-kB,[39] which may contribute to MDS transformation and to iron-mediated neoplasia, such as hepatoma.

An important, often neglected, mechanism of toxicity from iron overload is that of the increased risk of infection, which is the second commonest cause of death in TM. Several mechanisms come into play, the most important being transferrin saturation (TfS). This protein, in addition to its pivotal role in supplying iron to the erythron and other tissues, naturally exists where only an average of one-third of its 2 iron binding sites are occupied with Fe(III). A key role of transferrin is to deprive bacteria of the iron that these microorganisms require to grow. Although some bacteria have adapted to use transferrin iron, most have not, and so there is a paradigm shift in the availability of iron to microorganisms once transferrin becomes saturated. Other mechanisms, such as effects on neutrophil function have been postulated to be affected by TIO.[57] Recent work has shown that following blood transfusion, NTBI is liberated from the rapid catabolism of a proportion of nonviable red cells.[58] In principle, this and other forms of NTBI in plasma will be more available to microorganisms than transferrin iron.

DISTRIBUTION AND CONSEQUENCES OF TIO
Iron Distribution and Consequences in Thalassemia Major

The impact of chronic blood transfusion on body iron distribution is most completely described in TM, where transfusion typically begins in the first year of life. Transfused iron initially accumulates as storage iron in spleen, liver, and BM macrophages and later in hepatocytes, with 80% of storage iron in the liver. The storage capacity of the macrophage system following blood transfusion has not been recently studied, but historical sources estimate it at about 10 g. Histologic descriptions using Perl's stain show that with increasing TIO, increasing proportions are seen in hepatocytes once the macrophage system is saturated. Interestingly, particularly with optimal chelation therapy, TM patients today have low iron concentrations in hepatocytes, whereas macrophage iron remains present[59]; this contrasts with NTDT where iron accumulates through the portal system and concentrates in peri-portal hepatocytes with macrophage sparing. This distribution in NTDT is thought to be influenced further by low hepcidin levels, and therefore high macrophage ferroportin, due to high levels of IE typical in thalassemia.[59,60]

As TIO evolves, particularly with suboptimal chelation therapy, a variable proportion of iron 'escapes' from the liver into the endocrine tissues and heart. This gives rise to the classic pathology, morbidity, and mortality historically associated with TIO. An understanding of the effects of blood transfusion on body iron distribution is best appreciated from *post-mortem* data obtained during prechelation era,[61] because iron chelation fundamentally alters body iron distribution, being relatively tropic for hepatocellular iron compared with extrahepatic iron. Data obtained under these circumstances showed that in patients dying from complications of TIO, iron was unevenly distributed in the body, with high concentrations present in liver, heart, and endocrine tissues; very low in striated muscle; and none in the brain.[62] Remarkably, these patients typically died of heart failure in the second and third decades of life, although the myocardial iron concentration (MIC) was a fraction of that in the liver. This observation has recently been supported by magnetic resonance imaging (MRI) evidence[63]; examination of myocardial tissue both biochemically and by MRI at *post mortem* in patients dying from iron-induced cardiomyopathy showed an average MIC of only 5.98 ± 2.42 mg/g dw. Evidently, the heart is less adapted to accommodating high concentrations of storage iron than the liver, even though the storage iron is not directly toxic to cells (see later discussion).

Before the introduction of cardiac MRI monitoring and newer chelation regimens, the frequency of heart failure, diabetes, hypothyroidism, and hypoparathyroidism were all falling.[64] Hypogonadism (typically hypogonadotropic) is still an early and common feature of iron overload in TM, presenting with primary or secondary amenorrhea in women or poor growth and delayed puberty.[64] Since the introduction of cardiac MRI imaging and the intensification of chelation therapy in selected patients with increased MIC (mT2*<20 ms), the incidence of heart failure has fallen further. Indeed, in a recent cohort analysis of patients observed for a decade by cardiac MRI and receiving individually tailored chelation, heart failure was no longer the leading cause of death and the proportion of patients with myocardial iron (mT2*<20 ms) fell from 60% to 23%.[65] Cirrhosis, which develops 1 or 2 decades after heart failure, is becoming more common as patients live longer, being present in about 50% of patients at *post mortem* and is particularly common in patients with chronic hepatitis. Similarly, hepatocellular carcinoma[66] is becoming more common.

The relationship between the accumulation of liver iron and the risk of extrahepatic spread has been the source of intense debate. Early work suggested a close relationship in TM between the control of LIC with deferoxamine and long-term outcome from cardiomyopathy.[67] *Post-mortem* data in other diseases in the absence of chelation also suggested a relationship between transfusional ILR, LIC, and MIC.[68,69] When cardiac T2* became available in patients receiving a variety of chelation regimens, only a weak correlation between LIC and mT2* was seen, and it was argued therefore that control of LIC was not important to controlling MIC in TM and therefore to limiting potentially fatal cardiomyopathy.[70] The interpretation of the UCLH group was that this lack of correlation was mainly due to the high proportion of patients in this study having been on intensive chelation therapy with desferoxamine, which was subsequently shown to decrease LIC at a faster rate than myocardial iron[70,71]; this would therefore mask a potentially important relationship between these variables. Noetzli and colleagues[72] have somewhat clarified this issue by demonstrating the importance of longitudinal rather than cross-sectional analysis of the relationship. They showed that failure to control LIC over several years with chelation increased the risk of myocardial iron deposition. Conversely, LIC reduction had a delayed effect on decreasing the MIC. Longitudinal UK studies of the LVEF relationship to mT2* show that the risk of heart failure increases for mT2* less than 10 ms,[70] which approximates to MIC greater than 2.7 mg/g dw.[63] It can be concluded that LIC control in TM is important both to limiting liver damage and to controlling MIC, thus markedly reducing the risk of iron-mediated cardiomyopathy with heart failure.

Iron Distribution and Consequences in SCD

In patients receiving sufficient repeated transfusions to cause TIO, clinical consequences begin later than in TM, and thus effects on growth and sexual development are relatively uncommon. With transfusion, iron from erythrocyte catabolism initially accumulates in macrophages (Kupfer cells, sinusoidal compartment), but later, when the LIC exceeds 7 mg/g dw, in hepatocytes[73] (based on the Angelucci formula,[74] being equivalent to about 5 g of transfused iron in a 70 kg adult, or about 25 units of transfused blood). Hepatocellular iron stores in SCD only approached those of the sinusoidal compartment when total liver iron levels were high (>15 mg/g dw or about 50 units of transfused red cells).[73] Accumulation of liver iron without adequate chelation therapy risks fibrosis and cirrhosis.[75–77] Fibrosis has been reported as early as 2 years after initiation of transfusion and in about one-third of patients with LIC greater than 9 mg/g dw and in direct proportion to the LIC,[77] correlating with LIC[76] in the absence of hepatitis C infection.[77,78] The true frequency of cirrhosis in multitransfused adult SCD patients is not clear. *Post-mortem* studies found cirrhosis in 11% of all patients and in nearly half of patients who died with severe liver siderosis.[79]

The extrahepatic consequences of iron overload, particularly endocrine and cardiac effects, appear to be later or more delayed in SCD than TM. Myocardial iron deposition, as judged by T2* of less than 20 ms, is rare[80,81] and after more transfusion episodes in SCD than TM.[82] However, *post-mortem* studies show iron deposition in the heart in heavily transfused patients.[79] In SCD and TM patients matched for LIC, the incidence of heart disease, gonadal failure, and endocrine disturbances including growth delay, appear to be less for age less than 20 years in SCD.[83] Despite these differences from TM, SCD patients are unlikely to be completely protected from the extrahepatic effects of TIO and indeed cases of myocardial iron are reported by MRI.[84] Recent preliminary studies from the Multi Center Study of Iron Overload (MCSIO) group found evidence of increased pituitary iron in SCD with highest LIC.[85] In one study, patients with the lowest bone mass also had the highest serum iron values, although serum ferritin (SF) was within normal limits in these patients.[86] Furthermore there was an inverse correlation between the estimated pituitary iron and the pituitary volume, and hence its endocrine reserve. MRI may, in principle, identify early pituitary iron deposition in SCD before clinical manifestations are apparent.[85]

Increased iron has also been identified by MRI in the kidney.[87,88] This signal is highest in nontransfused patients with high levels of LDH, lacks correlation with LIC, and is higher than in TM patients, suggesting it originates from iron taken up by kidney from hemoglobin freed during intravascular hemolysis rather than iron delivered by transferrin or NTBI as a consequence of TIO. This signal also suggests that kidney R2* may be a biomarker for chronic hemolysis-mediated vascular complications in SCD. The extent to which this mechanism is implicated in renal damage in SCD is not clear.

Iron Distribution in Other Forms of TIO

TIO is seen in an increasing number of underlying conditions (**Table 1**). Iron accumulation in MDS may start even before patients become transfusion-dependent because of IE, which although variably counterbalanced by increased levels of cytokines upregulated during infections (eg, IL-6), may still inhibit hepcidin production[94] with subsequent increased iron absorption from the gut, as described earlier. Once transfusion begins, as with other forms of TIO, iron initially accumulates in RES and then in the liver. A key question with respect to the pathophysiology of iron overload is how rapidly iron spreads extrahepatically and how rapidly this is likely to be problematic and hence require chelation treatment. In the prechelation era, patients examined at *post-mortem* had an increased risk of myocardial iron with increasing numbers of blood transfusions.[68] Early studies with cardiac MRI showed increasing risk of myocardial iron as the number of transfusions exceeded 50 units.[95,96] Analysis of the relationship between transfusion and myocardial iron is complicated because patients have received chelation therapy in some but not all reports. Overall, in nonchelated MDS patients, iron spread to myocardium occurs after approximately 70 to 100 units of blood (containing 14–20 g iron).[68,95]

The prognostic impact of the resulting moderate degree of iron overload[94] for overall survival is not clear because it is difficult to clearly separate the effects of TIO from other comorbidities associated with BM failure without prospective controlled data. The prognostic importance of transfusion dependency for overall survival in patients with low- and intermediate-1-risk MDS has been examined in a retrospective analysis of European MDS and AML registry data,[97] which showed that patients with greater than 20 units transfused had a higher mortality rate (30%) within 2 years of diagnosis than transfusion-independent patients (5%). Among 705 patients followed for 2 years or until death, cardiac comorbidities were seen in 79% of chronically transfused patients versus only 54% of nontransfused MDS patients and 42% of a Medicare control population.[98] Although some retrospective data suggest a prognostic advantage to chelation therapy in MDS,[99–102] this has not yet been reported in prospective studies. It is clear that response with iron balance to chelation is similar to other forms of TIO. Improved hematopoiesis has been observed in 20% of patients receiving deferasirox for 1 year.[103] Responders showed a greater decrease in SF levels, suggesting that removal of iron from the BM plays a role in hematologic improvement.

There are a large number of disparate anemias that require chronic blood transfusion (see **Table 1**). Patient numbers reported are insufficient to draw clear conclusions about whether the risks of TIO differ from those of TM. DBA is perhaps the most common of the rare anemias, but this is a heterogeneous group of conditions with a presumed shared pathology of ribosomal protein dysfunction. Recent work by the MCSIO group suggests transfused DBA patients are particularly susceptible to the extrahepatic consequences of iron overload (Porter 2014, in preparation). The mechanisms and implications are discussed in the later discussion.

MECHANISMS UNDERLYING DISTRIBUTION OF TRANSFUSED IRON

Because the distribution of storage iron appears to be key to the pathophysiology of TIO, some of the putative mechanisms determining this distribution will be considered further.

Transferrin iron is delivered to tissues expressing TfR1 in a controlled way through receptor-mediated endocytosis. The expression of TfR and hence iron acquisition

Table 1
Conditions associated with transfusional iron overload

Condition	Underlying Mechanism for Iron Overload	Typical Distribution and Mechanism	Consequences
Inherited anemias			
Thalassemia major (TM)	Blood transfusions for anemia (+++) Increased iron absorption (+)	High NTBI (++) Liver, heart, endocrine	Cardiomyopathy Endocrinopathy Infection Cirrhosis, hepatoma
Sickle cell disease	Intermittent transfusion (++) Intravascular hemolysis with iron loss (+)	Liver predominantly High erythron iron utilization Low NTBI (+/−)	Cirrhosis (Extrahepatic iron)
Congenital dyserythropoietic anemia	Ineffective erythropoiesis Variable transfusion ∼10% of patients w CDA-I ∼5% with CDA-II <50% with other CDA variants	NTBI[89] (+)	Not systematically described
Sideroblastic anemia	Transfusion Ineffective erythropoiesis	Hepatic, myocardial High NTBI	Hepatic Myocardial[63,84]
Pyruvate kinase deficiency (severe)	Transfusion dependence Ineffective erythropoiesis Extravascular hemolysis	Like NTD unless transfused	Like NTDT unless transfused
Diamond Blackfan anemia (DBA)	Transfusion dependence (+++)	Hepatic and extrahepatic Low erythron iron utilization High NTBI (+++)	As with TM
Pure red cell aplasia	As above	As above	As above
Acquired anemias			
Aplastic anemia	Blood transfusions for anemia	Liver, heart, endocrine	Abnormal LFTs Heart[90] and liver failure[91] LIC reduced by chelation
Fanconi anemia	Regular transfusion	Not well described	As above
Myelodysplasias[92] (MDS)	Variable blood transfusion late onset Ineffective erythropoiesis (++)	Hepatic Extrahepatic >60–200 units	Hepatic[93] Cardiomyopathy[93] Infection
Myelofibrosis	High blood transfusion late onset Massive extravascular hemolysis	High LPI	Not described
Multiple myeloablative chemotherapies	Intermittent transfusion	Myocardial iron >100 units	Cardiomyopathy

from transferrin depends on iron homeostatic mechanisms (see earlier discussion). The erythron and hepatocytes are rich in these receptors as are cells undergoing proliferation where its expression is cell cycle dependent. As iron overload develops, transferrin becomes increasingly saturated, with the eventual appearance of NTBI, typically when TfS at greater than 75%.[104,105] The uptake of NTBI is less regulated than uptake from transferrin and the distribution is also substantially different.[106,107] This may account for the pattern of iron deposition and hence its toxicity in advanced TIO. In experimental models, NTBI is rapidly taken up by hepatocytes[108] and myocytes.[109] In cultured heart cells, NTBI species are taken up at 200 times the rate of transferrin iron and generate free radicals, lipid peroxidation, organelle dysfunction, and abnormal rhythmicity.[50,109] L-type calcium channels[106] and zinc transporters[110] have been implicated in NTBI uptake, which appears to be restricted to tissues known to accumulate iron. Plasma NTBI (or its subfractions) can also promote lipid peroxidation through the generation of free radicals[111] and associate with depletion of plasma antioxidants.[112]

The presumed relationship between NTBI levels and extrahepatic iron distribution has not been convincingly demonstrated clinically. A weak correlation between NTBI and mT2* was reported by Piga and colleagues[113] in TM patients. However, a careful analysis of NTBI levels in TM patients at UCLH has failed to find such an association (Garbowski, unpublished data, 2014), suggesting that the NTBI species heterogeneity may in principle affect the pattern of tissue iron uptake. NTBI species consist of iron citrate monomers, oligomers and polymers, as well as protein bound forms, and these may differ in their rates of uptake into tissues.[114,115] The various assays used to quantitate NTBI may measure different species that have variable importance to tissue iron uptake. It is not yet clear which assay is most appropriate to predicting extrahepatic iron distribution. The classic NTBI assay captures both directly chelatable iron, as well as a fraction of iron species that are only slowly chelatable.[115,116] Furthermore, the assay detects iron chelates of deferiprone[117] or deferasirox.[118] The labile plasma iron (LPI) assay measures a fraction of NTBI that is redoxactive and that is removed by the presence of iron chelators in plasma. The effect of iron chelate complexes is not clear but likely to affect this assay less than the NTBI assay. New assays for NTBI species are under development with the intention of obtaining an assay that has clear utility for predicting the risks of extrahepatic iron distribution.

A further reason why NTBI levels are difficult to link precisely to extrahepatic iron distribution is that NTBI is generated by factors other than iron overload. Two identified factors that generate NTBI are low levels of erythropoiesis and/or IE. Suppression of erythropoiesis, for example, following myeloablative chemotherapy, leads to decreased clearance of transferrin iron and the rapid appearance of NTBI,[119] which is quickly reversed following regeneration of erythropoiesis. In DBA, where recent work shows an absence of soluble transferrin receptors and hence of clearance of transferrin iron by the erythron, NTBI iron levels are particularly high and this condition is associated with a high propensity to myocardial iron accumulation (Porter 2014, in preparation). Conversely, a high utilization of transferrin iron such as in the highly expanded erythron in NTDT would desaturate small concentrations of transferrin, which in turn could inhibit NTBI iron uptake into target tissue. This effect would also be active in TM patients where the transfusion regimen does not completely suppress erythropoiesis. This hypothesis is currently under investigation (Garbowski 2014, in preparation).

Patients with SCD have low levels of NTBI[119,120] and LPI[121,122] compared with TM patients with similar levels of iron overload. It is an attractive hypothesis to link the low propensity for extrahepatic iron distribution in SCD to this observation. Of note, LPI is

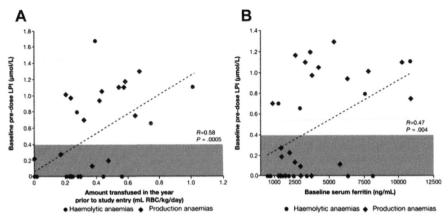

Fig. 2. (A) The relationship between baseline predose labile plasma iron (LPI) and transfusion rate in the year before study entry. There is a significant correlation (R = 0.58, P = .0005, n = 32) between transfusion rate in the year before study entry and baseline predose LPI in all patients. Hemolytic anemias are shown in circles and production anemias in diamonds. The gray area denotes the healthy reference range. (B) The relationship between baseline predose LPI and baseline serum ferritin (SF). There is a significant relationship (R = 0.47, P = .004) between baseline ferritin and baseline predose LPI for all patients. Hemolytic anemias are shown in circles and production anemias in diamonds. The gray area denotes the healthy reference range. (*From* Porter JB, Lin KH, Beris P, et al. Response of iron overload to deferasirox in rare transfusion-dependent anaemias: equivalent effects on SF and labile plasma iron for haemolytic or production anaemias. Eur J Haematol 2011;87(4):338–48. Copyright © 2011 John Wiley & Sons A/S.)

also low in SCD relative to other forms of TIO at similar levels of iron loading. However, patients with NTDT have high levels of NTBI[123,124] and LPI[125] but a very low risk of myocardial iron,[126] suggesting that absolute NTBI levels are not the only consideration. When a comparison of LPI in rare anemias resulting from hemolysis or from decreased red cell production was made,[127] both were associated with raised LPI, which was removed following chelation therapy. Analysis of the same patients showed a significant correlation of LPI levels with both the degree of iron overload (ferritin) and transfusional ILR (**Fig. 2**). This would support the notion that with increasing transfusional ILR, LPI and possibly the potential to extrahepatic iron loading increases. A systematic study of the relationship of transfusional loading rate, NTBI speciation, and extrahepatic complications of iron overload is warranted.

REFERENCES

1. Jacobs A. The pathology of iron overload. In: Jacobs A, Worwood M, editors. Iron in biochemistry and medicine. London: Academic Press; 1974. p. 427–59.
2. Bothwell T, Charlton RW, Cook JD, et al. Iron metabolism in man. Oxford (United Kingdom): Blackwell; 1979.
3. Nemeth E, Ganz T. Regulation of iron metabolism by hepcidin. Annu Rev Nutr 2006;26:323–42.
4. Mastrogiannaki M, Matak P, Keith B, et al. HIF-2alpha, but not HIF-1alpha, promotes iron absorption in mice. J Clin Invest 2009;119(5):1159–66.
5. Nemeth E, Tuttle MS, Powelson J, et al. Hepcidin regulates cellular iron efflux by binding to ferroportin and inducing its internalization. Science 2004;306(5704): 2090–3.

6. Delaby C, Pilard N, Goncalves AS, et al. Presence of the iron exporter ferroportin at the plasma membrane of macrophages is enhanced by iron loading and down-regulated by hepcidin. Blood 2005;106(12):3979–84.
7. Ganz T. Hepcidin and iron regulation, 10 years later. Blood 2011;117(17): 4425–33.
8. Darshan D, Anderson GJ. Interacting signals in the control of hepcidin expression. Biometals 2009;22(1):77–87.
9. Tanno T, Bhanu NV, Oneal PA, et al. High levels of GDF15 in thalassemia suppress expression of the iron regulatory protein hepcidin. Nat Med 2007;13(9): 1096–101.
10. Tanno T, Porayette P, Sripichai O, et al. Identification of TWSG1 as a second novel erythroid regulator of hepcidin expression in murine and human cells. Blood 2009;114(1):181–6.
11. Kautz L, Jung G, Valore EV, et al. Identification of erythroferrone as an erythroid regulator of iron metabolism, Nat Genet 2014. http://dx.doi.org/10.1038/ng. 2996.
12. Wilkins SJ, Frazer DM, Millard KN, et al. Iron metabolism in the hemoglobin-deficit mouse: correlation of diferric transferrin with hepcidin expression. Blood 2006;107(4):1659–64.
13. Nemeth E, Valore EV, Territo M, et al. Hepcidin, a putative mediator of anemia of inflammation, is a type II acute-phase protein. Blood 2002;14:14.
14. Pak M, Lopez MA, Gabayan V, et al. Suppression of hepcidin during anemia requires erythropoietic activity. Blood 2006;108(12):3730–5.
15. Frazer DM, Wilkins SJ, Darshan D, et al. Stimulated erythropoiesis with secondary iron loading leads to a decrease in hepcidin despite an increase in bone morphogenetic protein 6 expression. Br J Haematol 2012;157(5): 615–26.
16. Vokurka M, Krijt J, Sulc K, et al. Hepcidin mRNA levels in mouse liver respond to inhibition of erythropoiesis. Physiol Res 2006;55(6):667–74.
17. Lasocki S, Millot S, Andrieu V, et al. Phlebotomies or erythropoietin injections allow mobilization of iron stores in a mouse model mimicking intensive care anemia. Crit Care Med 2008;36(8):2388–94.
18. Rouault T, Stout C, Kaptain S, et al. Structural relationship between an iron-regulated RNA binding protein (IRE-BP) and aconitase: functional implications. Cell 1991;64:881–3.
19. Cooperman SS, Meyron-Holtz EG, Olivierre-Wilson H, et al. Microcytic anemia, erythropoietic protoporphyria, and neurodegeneration in mice with targeted deletion of iron-regulatory protein 2. Blood 2005;106(3):1084–91.
20. Taketani S. Aquisition, mobilization and utilization of cellular iron and heme: endless findings and growing evidence of tight regulation. Tohoku J Exp Med 2005;205(4):297–318.
21. De Domenico I, Ward DM, di Patti MC, et al. Ferroxidase activity is required for the stability of cell surface ferroportin in cells expressing GPI-ceruloplasmin. EMBO J 2007;26(12):2823–31.
22. Hider RC, Kong XL. Glutathione: a key component of the cytoplasmic labile iron pool. Biometals 2011;24(6):1179–87.
23. Porter J. Blood transfusion: quality and safety issues in thalassemia, basic requirements and new trends. Hemoglobin 2009;33(Suppl 1):S28–36.
24. Cazzola M, De Stefano P, Ponchio L, et al. Relationship between transfusion regimen and suppression of erythropoiesis in beta-thalassaemia major. Br J Haematol 1995;89(3):473–8.

25. Cazzola M, Borgna-Pignatti C, Locatelli F, et al. A moderate transfusion regimen may reduce iron loading in beta- thalassemia major without producing excessive expansion of erythropoiesis. Transfusion 1997;37(2):135–40.

26. Barry M, Flynn D, Letsky E, et al. Long term chelation therapy in thalassaemia: effect on liver iron concentration, liver histology and clinical progress. Br Med J 1974;2:16–20.

27. Koduri PR. Iron in sickle cell disease: a review why less is better. Am J Hematol 2003;73(1):59–63.

28. Sears DA, Anderson PR, Foy AL, et al. Urinary iron excretion and renal metabolism of hemoglobin in hemolytic diseases. Blood 1966;28(5):708–25.

29. Washington R, Boggs DR. Urinary iron in patients with sickle cell anamia. J Lab Clin Med 1975;86(1):17–23.

30. Keel SB, Doty RT, Yang Z, et al. A heme export protein is required for red blood cell differentiation and iron homeostasis. Science 2008;319(5864):825–8.

31. Porter JB, Walter PB, Neumayr LD, et al. Mechanisms of plasma NTBI generation: insights from comparing transfused diamond blackfan anaemia with sickle cell and thalassaemia patients. Br J Haematol, in press.

32. Adams RJ, Brambilla D. Discontinuing prophylactic transfusions used to prevent stroke in sickle cell disease. N Engl J Med 2005;353(26):2769–78.

33. Vichinsky E, Bernaudin F, Forni GL, et al. Long-term safety and efficacy of deferasirox (exjade®) in transfused patients with sickle cell disease treated for up to 5 years. Br J Haematol 2011;154:387–97.

34. Porter JB, Huehns ER. Transfusion and exchange transfusion in sickle cell anaemias, with particular reference to iron metabolism. Acta Haematol 1987;78(2–3): 198–205.

35. Kim HC, Dugan NP, Silber JH, et al. Erythrocytapheresis therapy to reduce iron overload in chronically transfused patients with sickle cell disease. Blood 1994; 83:1136–42.

36. Porter J, Galanello R, Saglio G, et al. Relative response of patients with myelodysplastic syndromes and other transfusion-dependent anaemias to deferasirox (ICL670): a 1-yr prospective study. Eur J Haematol 2008;80(2):168–76.

37. Porter JB. Pathophysiology of iron overload. Hematol Oncol Clin North Am 2005; 19(Suppl 1):7–12.

38. Zuo Y, Xiang B, Yang J, et al. Oxidative modification of caspase-9 facilitates its activation via disulfide-mediated interaction with Apaf-1. Cell Res 2009;19(4): 449–57.

39. Aggarwal BB. Nuclear factor-kappaB: the enemy within. Cancer Cell 2004;6(3): 203–8.

40. Ceccarelli D, Gallesi D, Giovannini F, et al. Relationship between free iron level and rat liver mitochondrial dysfunction in experimental dietary iron overload. Biochem Biophys Res Commun 1995;209(1):53–9.

41. Breuer W, Epsztejn S, Millgram P, et al. Transport of iron and other transition metals into cells as revealed by a fluorescent probe. Am J Physiol 1995; 268(6 Pt 1):C1354–61.

42. Cooper CE, Lynagh GR, Hoyes KP, et al. The relationship of intracellular iron chelation to the inhibition and regeneration of human ribonucleotide reductase. J Biol Chem 1996;271(34):20291–9.

43. Cooper CE, Porter JB. Ribonucleotide reductase, lipoxygenase and the intracellular low- molecular-weight iron pool. Biochem Soc Trans 1997;25(1):75–80.

44. Galaris D, Skiada V, Barbouti A. Redox signaling and cancer: the role of "labile" iron. Cancer Lett 2008;266(1):21–9.

45. Epsztejn S, Glickstein H, Picard V, et al. H-ferritin subunit overexpression in erythroid cells reduces the oxidative stress response and induces multidrug resistance properties. Blood 1999;94(10):3593–603.
46. Marx JJM, van Asbeck BS. Use of chelators in preventing hydroxyl radical damage: adult respiratory distress syndrome as an experimental model for the treatment of oxygen-radical-mediated tissue damage. Acta Haematol 1996;95:49–62.
47. Kornbrust DJ, Mavis RD. Microsomal lipid peroxidation. 1. Characterisation of the role of iron and NADPH. Mol Pharmacol 1980;17:400–7.
48. Bacon BR, Tavill AS, Brittenham GM, et al. Hepatic lipid peroxidation in vivo in rats with chronic iron overload. J Clin Invest 1983;71(3):429–39.
49. Myers BM, Prendergast FG, Holman R, et al. Alterations in the structure, physicochemical properties, and pH of hepatocyte lysosomes in experimental iron overload. J Clin Invest 1991;88(4):1207–15.
50. Link G, Pinson A, Hershko C. Iron loading of cultured cardiac myocytes modifies sarcolemmal structure and increases lysosomal fragility. J Lab Clin Med 1993; 121(1):127–34.
51. Link G, Saada A, Pinson A, et al. Mitochondrial respiratory enzymes are a major target of iron toxicity in rat heart cells. J Lab Clin Med 1998;131(5): 466–74.
52. Zhao M, Laissue JA, Zimmermann A. Hepatocyte apoptosis in hepatic iron overload diseases. Histol Histopathol 1997;12(2):367–74.
53. Jacob AK, Hotchkiss RS, Swanson PE, et al. Injection of iron compounds followed by induction of the stress response causes tissue injury and apoptosis. Shock 2000;14(4):460–4.
54. Houglum K, Filip M, Witztum JL, et al. Malondialdehyde and 4-hydroxynonenal protein adducts in plasma and liver of rats with iron overload. J Clin Invest 1990; 86(6):1991–8.
55. Parola M, Pinzani A, Casini E, et al. Stimulation of lipid peroxidation or 4-hydroxynonenal treatment increased procollagen (I) gene expression in human fat storing cells. J Biol Chem 1993;264:16957–62.
56. Bissell DM, Wang SS, Jarnagin WR, et al. Cell specific expression of transforming growth factor-ß in the rat liver. J Clin Invest 1995;96:447–55.
57. Hoepelman IM, Bezemer WA, van Doornmalen E, et al. Lipid peroxidation of human granulocytes (PMN) and monocytes by iron complexes. Br J Haematol 1989;72(4):584–8.
58. Hod EA, Zhang N, Sokol SA, et al. Transfusion of red blood cells after prolonged storage produces harmful effects that are mediated by iron and inflammation. Blood 2010;115(21):4284–92.
59. Origa R, Galanello R, Ganz T, et al. Liver iron concentrations and urinary hepcidin in beta-thalassemia. Haematologica 2007;92(5):583–8.
60. Kattamis A, Papassotiriou I, Palaiologou D, et al. The effects of erythropoetic activity and iron burden on hepcidin expression in patients with thalassemia major. Haematologica 2006;91(6):809–12.
61. Modell B. Management of thalassaemia major. Br Med Bull 1976;32(3):270–6.
62. Modell B, Matthews R. Thalassemia in Britain and Australia. Birth Defects Orig Artic Ser 1976;12(8):13–29.
63. Carpenter JP, He T, Kirk P, et al. On T2* magnetic resonance and cardiac iron. Circulation 2011;123(14):1519–28.
64. Borgna-Pignatti C, Rugolotto S, De Stefano P, et al. Survival and complications in patients with thalassemia major treated with transfusion and deferoxamine. Haematologica 2004;89(10):1187–93.

65. Thomas AS, Garbowski M, Ang AL, et al. A decade follow-up of a thalassemia major (TM) cohort monitored by cardiac magnetic resonance imaging (CMR): significant reduction in patients with cardiac iron and in total mortality. Blood 2010;116(21):1011.

66. Borgna-Pignatti C, Vergine G, Lombardo T, et al. Hepatocellular carcinoma in the thalassaemia syndromes. Br J Haematol 2004;124(1):114–7.

67. Brittenham GM, Griffith PM, Nienhuis AW, et al. Efficacy of deferoxamine in preventing complications of iron overload in patients with thalassemia major. N Engl J Med 1994;331(9):567–73.

68. Buja LM, Roberts WC. Iron in the heart. Etiology and clinical significance. Am J Med 1971;51(2):209–21.

69. St Pierre TG, Tran KC, Webb J, et al. Organ-specific crystalline structures of ferritin cores in beta-thalassemia/hemoglobin E. Biol Met 1991;4(3):162–5.

70. Anderson LJ, Holden S, Davis B, et al. Cardiovascular T2-star (T2*) magnetic resonance for the early diagnosis of myocardial iron overload. Eur Heart J 2001;22(23):2171–9.

71. Anderson LJ, Westwood MA, Holden S, et al. Myocardial iron clearance during reversal of siderotic cardiomyopathy with intravenous desferrioxamine: a prospective study using T2* cardiovascular magnetic resonance. Br J Haematol 2004;127(3):348–55.

72. Noetzli LJ, Carson SM, Nord AS, et al. Longitudinal analysis of heart and liver iron in thalassemia major. Blood 2008;112(7):2973–8.

73. Hankins JS, Smeltzer MP, McCarville MB, et al. Patterns of liver iron accumulation in patients with sickle cell disease and thalassemia with iron overload. Eur J Haematol 2010;85(1):51–7.

74. Angelucci E, Brittenham GM, McLaren CE, et al. Hepatic iron concentration and total body iron stores in thalassemia major. N Engl J Med 2000;343(5):327–31.

75. Comer GM, Ozick LA, Sachdev RK, et al. Transfusion-related chronic liver disease in sickle cell anemia. Am J Gastroenterol 1991;86(9):1232–4.

76. Harmatz P, Butensky E, Quirolo K, et al. Severity of iron overload in patients with sickle cell disease receiving chronic red blood cell transfusion therapy. Blood 2000;96(1):76–9.

77. Olivieri NF. Progression of iron overload in sickle cell disease. Semin Hematol 2001;38(1 Suppl 1):57–62.

78. Brown K, Subramony C, May W, et al. Hepatic iron overload in children with sickle cell anemia on chronic transfusion therapy. J Pediatr Hematol Oncol 2009;31(5):309–12.

79. Darbari DS, Kple-Faget P, Kwagyan J, et al. Circumstances of death in adult sickle cell disease patients. Am J Hematol 2006;81(11):858–63.

80. Porter JB. Concepts and goals in the management of transfusional iron overload. Am J Hematol 2007;82(Suppl 12):1136–9.

81. Westwood MA, Shah F, Anderson LJ, et al. Myocardial tissue characterization and the role of chronic anemia in sickle cell cardiomyopathy. J Magn Reson Imaging 2007;26(3):564–8.

82. Wood JC, Tyszka JM, Carson S, et al. Myocardial iron loading in transfusion-dependent thalassemia and sickle cell disease. Blood 2004;103(5):1934–6.

83. Vichinsky E, Butensky E, Fung E, et al. Comparison of organ dysfunction in transfused patients with SCD or beta thalassemia. Am J Hematol 2005;80(1):70–4.

84. Glanville J, Eleftheriou P, Porter J. MRI evidence of cardiac iron accumulation in myelodysplasia and unusual anemias. Blood 2006;108(11):446a [abstract: 1553].

85. Wang ZJ, Wood J, Walter P, et al. Iron distribution assessed by MRI in sickle cell disease, thalassemia and diamond blackfan anemia (MSCIO pilot study). Am J Hematol 2013;88(5):E96.
86. Sadat-Ali M, Sultan O, Al-Turki H, et al. Does high serum iron level induce low bone mass in sickle cell anemia? Biometals 2011;24(1):19–22.
87. Schein A, Enriquez C, Coates TD, et al. Magnetic resonance detection of kidney iron deposition in sickle cell disease: a marker of chronic hemolysis. J Magn Reson Imaging 2008;28(3):698–704.
88. Vasavda N, Gutierrez L, House MJ, et al. Renal iron load in sickle cell disease is influenced by severity of haemolysis. Br J Haematol 2012;157(5):599–605.
89. Wickramasinghe SN, Thein SL, Srichairatanakool S, et al. Determinants of iron status and bilirubin levels in congenital dyserythropoietic anaemia type I. Br J Haematol 1999;107(3):522–5.
90. Ohnuma K, Toyoda Y, Nishihira H, et al. Detection of early cardiac dysfunction in patients with transfusion-dependent aplastic anemia and chronic iron overload in childhood. Stress-velocity relation as a sensitive index by echocardiography. Rinsho Ketsueki 1996;37(9):825–32 [in Japanese].
91. Kim KH, Kim JW, Rhee JY, et al. Cost analysis of iron-related complications in a single institute. Korean J Intern Med 2009;24(1):33–6.
92. Takatoku M, Uchiyama T, Okamoto S, et al. Retrospective nationwide survey of Japanese patients with transfusion-dependent MDS and aplastic anemia highlights the negative impact of iron overload on morbidity/mortality. Eur J Haematol 2007;78(6):487–94.
93. Lee JW. Iron chelation therapy in the myelodysplastic syndromes and aplastic anemia: a review of experience in South Korea. Int J Hematol 2008;88(1):16–23.
94. Santini V, Girelli D, Sanna A, et al. Hepcidin levels and their determinants in different types of myelodysplastic syndromes. PLoS One 2011;6(8):e23109.
95. Jensen PD, Jensen FT, Christensen T, et al. Evaluation of myocardial iron by magnetic resonance imaging during iron chelation therapy with deferrioxamine: indication of close relation between myocardial iron content and chelatable iron pool. Blood 2003;101(11):4632–9.
96. Jaeger M, Aul C, Sohngen D, et al. Secondary hemochromatosis in polytransfused patients with myelodysplastic syndromes. Beitr Infusionsther 1992;30:464–8 [in German].
97. de Swart L, Smith A, Fenaux P, et al. Transfusion-dependency is the most important prognostic factor for survival in 1000 newly diagnosed MDS patients with low- and intermediate-1 risk MDS in the European leukemianet MDS registry. Blood 2011;118(21):2775.
98. Goldberg SL, Chen E, Corral M, et al. Incidence and clinical complications of myelodysplastic syndromes among United States medicare beneficiaries. J Clin Oncol 2010;28(17):2847–52.
99. Leitch HA, Leger CS, Goodman TA, et al. Improved survival in patients with myelodysplastic syndrome receiving iron chelation therapy. Hematological Oncology 2010;28(1):40–8.
100. Rose C, Brechignac S, Vassilief D, et al. Does iron chelation therapy improve survival in regularly transfused lower risk MDS patients? A multicenter study by the GFM. Leuk Res 2010;34(7):864–70.
101. Fox F, Kundgen A, Nachtkamp K, et al. Matched-pair analysis of 186 MDS patients receiving iron chelation therapy or transfusion therapy only. Blood 2009;114(22):1747.

102. Komrokji RS, Ali NH, Padron E, et al. Impact of iron chelation therapy on overall survival and AML transformation in lower risk MDS patients treated at the Moffitt Cancer Center. Blood 2011;118(21):2776.

103. Gattermann N, Finelli C, Della Porta M, et al. Hematologic responses to deferasirox therapy in transfusion-dependent patients with myelodysplastic syndromes. Haematologica 2012;97(9):1364–71.

104. Le Lan C, Loreal O, Cohen T, et al. Redox active plasma iron in C282Y/C282Y hemochromatosis. Blood 2005;105(11):4527–31.

105. Loreal O, Gosriwatana I, Guyader D, et al. Determination of non-transferrin-bound iron in genetic hemochromatosis using a new HPLC-based method. J Hepatol 2000;32(5):727–33.

106. Oudit GY, Sun H, Trivieri MG, et al. L-type Ca2+ channels provide a major pathway for iron entry into cardiomyocytes in iron-overload cardiomyopathy. Nat Med 2003;9(9):1187–94.

107. Oudit GY, Trivieri MG, Khaper N, et al. Role of L-type Ca2+ channels in iron transport and iron-overload cardiomyopathy. J Mol Med 2006;84(5):349–64.

108. Brissot P, Wright TL, Ma WL, et al. Efficient clearance of non-transferrin-bound iron by rat liver. Implications for hepatic iron loading in iron overload states. J Clin Invest 1985;76(4):1463–70.

109. Link G, Pinson A, Kahane I, et al. Iron loading modifies the fatty acid composition of cultured rat myocardial cells and liposomal vesicles: effect of ascorbate and alpha-tocopherol on myocardial lipid peroxidation. J Lab Clin Med 1989; 114:243–9.

110. Liuzzi JP, Aydemir F, Nam H, et al. Zip14 (Slc39a14) mediates non-transferrin-bound iron uptake into cells. Proc Natl Acad Sci U S A 2006;103(37):13612–7.

111. Gutteridge J, Rowley D, Griffiths E, et al. Low molecular weight iron complexes and oxygen radical reactions in idiopathic haemochromatosis. Clin Sci 1985;68: 463–7.

112. De Luca C, Filosa A, Grandinetti M, et al. Blood antioxidant status and urinary levels of catecholamine metabolites in beta-thalassemia. Free Radic Res 1999;30(6):453–62.

113. Piga A, Longo F, Duca L, et al. High nontransferrin bound iron levels and heart disease in thalassemia major. Am J Hematol 2009;84(1):29–33.

114. Grootveld M, Bell JD, Halliwell B, et al. Non-transferrin-bound iron in plasma or serum from patients with idiopathic hemochromatosis. Characterization by high performance liquid chromatography and nuclear magnetic resonance spectroscopy. J Biol Chem 1989;264(8):4417–22.

115. Evans RW, Rafique R, Zarea A, et al. Nature of non-transferrin-bound iron: studies on iron citrate complexes and thalassemic sera. J Biol Inorg Chem 2008;13(1):57–74.

116. Evans P, Kayyali R, Hider RC, et al. Mechanisms for the shuttling of plasma non-transferrin-bound iron (NTBI) onto deferoxamine by deferiprone. Transl Res 2010;156(2):55–67.

117. Aydinok Y, Evans P, Manz CY, et al. Timed non-transferrin bound iron determinations probe the origin of chelatable iron pools during deferiprone regimens and predict chelation response. Haematologica 2012;97(6):835–41.

118. Lal A, Porter J, Sweeters N, et al. Combined chelation therapy with deferasirox and deferoxamine in thalassemia. Blood Cells Mol Dis 2013;50(2):99–104.

119. Shah F, Westwood MA, Evans PJ, et al. Discordance in MRI assessment of iron distribution and plasma NTBI between transfusionally iron loaded adults with sickle cell and thalassaemia syndromes. Blood 2002;100:468a.

120. Walter PB, Fung EB, Killilea DW, et al. Oxidative stress and inflammation in iron-overloaded patients with beta-thalassaemia or sickle cell disease. Br J Haematol 2006;135(2):254–63.
121. Koren A, Fink D, Admoni O, et al. Non-transferrin-bound labile plasma iron and iron overload in sickle-cell disease: a comparative study between sickle-cell disease and beta-thalassemic patients. Eur J Haematol 2010;84(1):72–8.
122. Ghoti H, Goitein O, Koren A, et al. No evidence for myocardial iron overload and free iron species in multitransfused patients with sickle/beta-thalassaemia. Eur J Haematol 2010;84(1):59–63.
123. Taher A, Musallam KM, El Rassi F, et al. Levels of non-transferrin-bound iron as an index of iron overload in patients with thalassaemia intermedia. Br J Haematol 2009;146(5):569–72.
124. Porter J, Cappellini CM, Kattamis A, et al. Relationships between plasma non-transferrin-bound iron and markers of iron overload, anaemia and ineffective erythropoiesis in non-transfusion-dependent thalassaemia syndromes. Haematologica 2011;96:228. [abstract: #0536].
125. Pootrakul P, Breuer W, Sametband M, et al. Labile plasma iron (LPI) as an indicator of chelatable plasma redox activity in iron-overloaded beta-thalassemia/HbE patients treated with an oral chelator. Blood 2004;104(5):1504–10.
126. Origa R, Barella S, Argiolas GM, et al. No evidence of cardiac iron in 20 never- or minimally-transfused patients with thalassemia intermedia. Haematologica 2008;93(7):1095–6.
127. Porter JB, Lin KH, Beris P, et al. Response of iron overload to deferasirox in rare transfusion-dependent anaemias: equivalent effects on serum ferritin and labile plasma iron for haemolytic or production anaemias. Eur J Haematol 2011;87(4):338–48.

Transfusional Iron Overload and Iron Chelation Therapy in Thalassemia Major and Sickle Cell Disease

CrossMark

Maria Marsella, MD, Caterina Borgna-Pignatti, MD*

KEYWORDS

- Thalassemia major • Sickle cell disease • Iron overload • Iron chelation
- Deferoxamine • Deferiprone • Deferasirox

KEY POINTS

- Thalassemia major is caused by defects in the synthesis of one or more of the globin sub-units of hemoglobin, resulting in variable phenotypes.
- The yearly incidence of symptomatic individuals is estimated at 1 in 100,000 people throughout the world (22,989 new births) and 1 in 10,000 people in the European Union.
- Patients with thalassemia, being transfusion-dependent and having a hyperactive marrow, accumulate iron in tissues.
- The worldwide birth rate of individuals with symptomatic sickle cell disease (SCD) is approximately 2.2 per 1000 births. However, the disease incidence varies between ethnic groups.
- Blood transfusions may be required in both acute and chronic complications of SCD.
- SCD and thalassemia major differ in iron-loading patterns and in the prevalence of iron-induced organ damage.

 Video demonstrating a schedule of administration of iron chelators accompanies this article at http://www.hemonc.theclinics.com/

INTRODUCTION

The natural history of both thalassemia major (TM) and sickle cell disease (SCD) has been completely transformed in industrialized countries by the introduction of modern blood transfusions (filtered red cell concentrates that carry an extremely low residual

Disclosure: C. Borgna-Pignatti has received speaker's honoraria from Apopharma and Novartis. M. Marsella reports no conflicts of interest.
Department of Medical Sciences, University of Ferrara, Azienda Ospedale-Università Via Aldo Moro 8, Cona, Ferrara, Italy
* Corresponding author.
E-mail address: c.borgna@unife.it

Hematol Oncol Clin N Am 28 (2014) 703–727
http://dx.doi.org/10.1016/j.hoc.2014.04.004
0889-8588/14/$ – see front matter © 2014 Elsevier Inc. All rights reserved.

risk of pathogen transmission) and iron chelation. The life expectancy in TM has changed from a few years to 5 or 6 decades and it may soon equal that of the nonthalassemic population. Mortality continues to decrease, mainly because of a reduction in cardiac deaths (**Fig. 1**).

Despite the difficulties they still encounter, patients with SCD have also experienced great improvement in quality of life thanks to the introduction of transfusions and hydroxyurea for the prevention and treatment of several complications.[1–4]

BLOOD TRANSFUSIONS
TM

The anemia of TM becomes symptomatic between 6 months and 2 years of age, requiring the institution of a regular transfusion program. As a consequence of continuous anemia, erythropoiesis, although inefficient, can be intense; the bone marrow undergoes an enormous expansion with consequent distortion of facial features, and the plasma volume increases. In addition, hepatosplenomegaly develops. A regimen maintaining a minimum hemoglobin concentration of 9.5 to 10.5 g/dL prevents all the above complications and fosters normal growth at least until puberty.

SCD

Red blood cell transfusions are a mainstay in the treatment of both acute and chronic SCD complications.[5,6] Most patients receive at least one transfusion in their lifetime, usually for acute complications. Blood transfusions increase arterial oxygen pressure and hemoglobin oxygen-affinity, thereby reducing red cell sickling, and they also improve microvascular perfusion.[7,8] Regular blood transfusion regimens additionally suppress endogenous erythropoiesis and therefore the production of red cells containing sickle hemoglobin.

Common indications for both acute and chronic transfusions are shown in **Box 1**.[9]

Erythrocytapheresis in SCD

In SCD, erythrocytapheresis or manual exchange transfusions are alternatives to long-term simple transfusions. Automated erythrocytapheresis is the most accurate method for achieving a target hemoglobin S, but it is also expensive, invasive, and not available in all centers. Manual partial exchange transfusion can be used as an alternative. Both methods slow or prevent further accumulation of transfusional iron.[26]

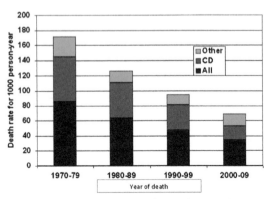

Fig. 1. Death rate of patients with TM observed in Italy according to cause and year of death. CD, cardiac disease.

Box 1
Common indications for both acute and chronic transfusions

Indications for acute transfusions

- After surgery and/or general anesthesia[10,11]
- Acute splenic or hepatic sequestration[12,13]
- Aplastic crisis[14]
- Acute chest syndrome[a,15,16]
- Stroke or acute neurologic deficit[a,17,18]
- Multiorgan failure[a,19]

Indications for regular transfusion programs

- Primary and secondary stroke prevention[20,21]
- Recurrent acute chest syndrome[22–24]
- Progressive organ failure[25]

  [a] May require exchange transfusion.

IRON OVERLOAD

Transfusional iron intake amounts to approximately 0.3 to 0.5 mg/kg/d for most patients.[27] The transfusion iron burden can be calculated as the total amount of pure red blood cells transfused (volume of packed red cells multiplied by the hematocrit [%] of the unit) $\times$ 1.08.[28] Most units of transfused red cells contain 180 to 200 mg of iron.

Part of the non-transferrin-bound iron circulating in the plasma (labile plasma iron) produces reactive radicals, and the resulting oxidation products are thought to be responsible for a large part of the iron accumulation and parenchymal cell injury associated with regular transfusions.[29] The organs particularly affected are the heart, liver, pancreas, and endocrine glands.

Based on the experience collected in hereditary hemochromatosis, a liver iron concentration (LIC) of 7 mg/g was considered compatible with a normal life expectancy and therefore an appropriate target for control of iron overload with chelation therapy.[30] Today, however, on the basis of numerous studies of magnetic resonance imaging (MRI), it is clear that the LIC does not consistently reflect the cardiac iron content and therefore cannot accurately predict prognosis. Without effective iron chelation, death commonly occurs in the second or third decade in patients with TM, usually because of iron-induced cardiac disease.

Does Iron Overload Differ Between SCD and TM?

Iron metabolism, and consequently, patterns of iron loading differ in SCD and TM. Erythropoiesis is variably increased in SCD, but it is not ineffective. Unlike patients with thalassemia, patients with nontransfused SCD do not develop systemic iron overload because of increased iron absorption, and they may actually present iron deficiency, possibly related to intravascular hemolysis and the resulting excessive urinary loss of iron.[31]

Inflammation, which is part of the pathophysiology of SCD, increases synthesis of hepcidin and consequently decreases iron absorption and enhances retention of iron within the reticulo-endothelial system. As a result, tissues and organs affected by iron overload are different in SCD and TM.[32,33] Specifically, iron-induced cardiac and endocrine dysfunction is less common in SCD.

Transfusion regimens may sometimes differ in the 2 populations. Patients with TM may require transfusions every 2 to 4 weeks to maintain hemoglobin values between 9 and 10 g/dL, beginning at a very young age (3–6 months). On the other hand, in SCD regular transfusions are usually started later in life, and many patients, particularly adults, receive occasional simple transfusions rather than transfusions on a regular schedule.

Iron-induced Organ Damage in SCD

As noted above, organ damage secondary to iron overload has been found to be disease-specific. In a retrospective study, Vichinsky and colleagues[34] reported a higher prevalence of cardiac disease (20% vs 0%), growth failure (27% vs 9%), and endocrine failure (37% vs 0%) in 30 patients with TM compared with 43 patients with SCD. In a multivariate analysis, the only significant predictors of combined endocrine and cardiac disease were duration of chronic transfusion and diagnosis.

Oxidative stress also differs in the 2 diseases. A study investigated the relationship between iron overload and disease-specific organ damage in TM and SCD by analyzing biomarkers of oxidative stress, inflammation, and tissue injury. Inflammation in SCD induced higher levels of the anti-oxidant γ-tocopherol compared with TM, leading to decreased tissue peroxidation and injury.[33]

Complications of Iron Overload

Heart

Cardiac problems are a frequent consequence of iron overload and in particular of the peroxidative damage to lysosomes and mitochondria by the labile iron pool. A recent Italian cooperative study demonstrated that 22% of patients with TM undergoing MRI had one or more cardiac problems, including heart dysfunction (66%), arrhythmias (14%), and both heart dysfunction and arrhythmias (19%).[35] The prevalence of cardiac disease was significantly higher in male than in female patients (**Fig. 2**) and was dependent on the cohort of birth. Heart failure and arrhythmias have been responsible for more than 70% of all deaths (**Fig. 3**).[36–39] An expert consensus from the American Heart Association on the diagnosis and treatment of cardiac dysfunction in TM has been recently issued.[40]

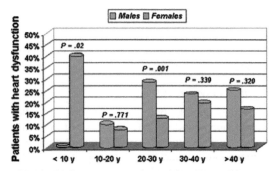

Fig. 2. Percentage of heart dysfunction in male and female patients according to age. The difference between sexes was statistically significant in the third decade. (*From* Marsella M, Borgna-Pignatti C, Meloni A, et al. Cardiac iron and cardiac disease in males and females with transfusion-dependent thalassemia major: a T2* magnetic resonance imaging study. Haematologica 2011;96(4):515–20.)

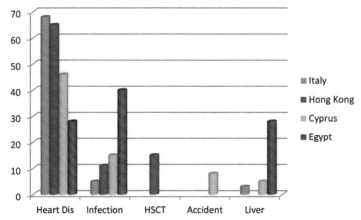

Fig. 3. Most common causes of death among patients with TM in 4 countries. HSCT, hemopoietic stem cell transplantation.

Increasing literature suggests that patients with SCD may be protected from iron-related cardiac damage.[34,41,42] Several MRI studies demonstrated an absence of cardiac iron in patients with SCD. Wood and colleagues[43] found that heavily iron-loaded patients with SCD had normal cardiac T2* values despite monthly transfusions for an average of 9.3 years. More recently, similar findings were described in 23 Lebanese patients with SCD (mean cardiac T2* = 37.3 ± 6.2 ms; range: 21.9–46.8 ms), even in the presence of significant systemic and hepatic iron overload.[41] However, in regularly transfused patients with SCD, effective chelation therapy is still needed to avoid hepatic iron overload and iron-related organ dysfunction.

Liver
Liver iron overload is a cause of fibrosis and cirrhosis, especially when associated with blood-transmitted hepatotropic viruses, in particular HCV.[44] Cirrhosis is a major risk factor for liver failure and can evolve to hepatocellular carcinoma.[45] The prevalence of cirrhosis in patients with TM ranges from 10% to 20%.[46] However, as described earlier, the LIC does not always correlate well with cardiac iron and should therefore not be used alone to predict risk for iron-related cardiac disease.[47]

The hepatic pattern of iron distribution differs in patients with SCD compared with patients with TM. In a recent histologic study, patients with SCD were found to have significantly less hepatic fibrosis and inflammation at similar levels of LIC as patients with TM. Although patients with SCD had predominantly sinusoidal iron deposition, parenchymal iron deposition was observed even at low LIC.[48] Iron-related hepatic damage in patients with SCD may also be enhanced by the high incidence of transfusion-acquired hepatitis C in some developing countries.[49–51]

Endocrine organs
In TM, iron deposition and structural damage of the pancreas the pituitary, parathyroid, thyroid, and adrenal glands and the gonads have been demonstrated histologically and by MRI. The reported prevalence of endocrine complications in TM is shown in **Fig. 4**.

Despite iron overload, endocrinopathies are less frequent in SCD. A study comparing iron overloaded subjects with TM and SCD confirmed a higher prevalence of endocrinopathies in patients with TM. Moreover, the rate of endocrine disorders was similar in transfused and nontransfused patients with SCD, suggesting a role of the disease in modulating iron-related endocrine injury.[52]

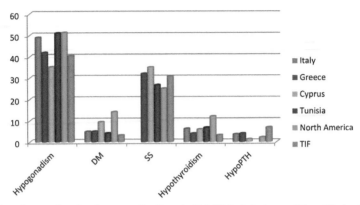

Fig. 4. Prevalence of endocrine complications in TM. DM, diabetes mellitus; SS, short stature; TIF, Thalassemia International Federation.

IRON CHELATION

To prevent hemosiderosis, iron must be chelated and excreted. Successful long-term iron chelation therapy depends on the achievement of neutral or negative iron balance, meaning the amount of iron excreted with chelation therapy must be the same or more than the amount of iron acquired from transfusion and gastrointestinal absorption. Because the mean iron intake differs even among patients with the same hematologic disorder because of factors such as molecular defect, presence of red cell alloantibodies, spleen size, and other factors, it is important to know the actual transfusional iron intake for a patient when choosing the dose of chelator.[53] Three iron chelators are now commercially available (**Tables 1** and **2**) and a fourth is undergoing phase 3 trials (**Box 2**).

Deferoxamine B

DFO, a hydroxamic acid and hexadentate chelator, was developed over 50 years ago as the first available chelating agent (**Box 3**). It did not undergo the formal trials that would currently be required before being approved by the regulatory agencies. The extraordinary effect of the introduction of chelation in clinical practice is demonstrated by the change in survival of patients with TM subdivided by cohort of birth. In fact, a very marked improvement was seen for patients born after 1974 who had the benefit of subcutaneous chelation from the first years of life.[36] Treatment with continuous intravenous DFO has been shown to improve myocardial iron, even in the most overloaded hearts with average myocardial T2* values of less than 6 ms, and to rescue patients in congestive heart failure.[83] The main limit of DFO is the inconvenience of parenteral administration. The patients' compliance, therefore, is often erratic, especially during the teenage years.

Twice daily subcutaneous bolus injections induce the same urinary iron excretion as the pump-mediated, continuous infusions and are often well accepted by older patients. This approach also represents an alternative where pumps are not available.[84–86]

Deferiprone

Deferiprone (DFP) is a member of the family of the hydroxypyridin-4-one chelators (**Box 4**). Three molecules of DFP are required to fully bind the 6 coordination sites of an iron atom, after having been glucuronidated in the liver.

DFP binds iron in both parenchymal and reticulo-endothelial cells and is excreted in the urine within 3 to 4 hours and therefore it must be administered every 8 hours. Use in children has been reported from India,[89] Egypt,[90] Greece,[91] and Thailand.[92] A multi-center international study to analyze the safety and efficacy of DFP in the pediatric population is underway. This study is the first large randomized controlled trial comparing the 2 oral chelators, DFP and deferasirox (DFX).[93] Voskaridou and colleagues[94] reported a statistically significant decrease in serum ferritin levels in 10 of 15 patients with SCD and improvement of liver T2 values in 8 of 12 patients, after 12 months of therapy with DFP. Several studies have demonstrated increased effectiveness of DFP in comparison to DFO in removing cardiac iron, resulting in reduced morbidity and mortality.[45,95–97] In a randomized controlled trial, DFP monotherapy was significantly more effective than DFO over 1 year in improving myocardial T2* and left ventricular ejection fraction.[98] Other MRI results have shown lower levels of cardiac iron as measured by T2* in DFP-treated patients.[99]

Deferasirox

The safety and efficacy of DFX are similar in pediatric and adult patients with TM (**Box 5**).[74] DFX seems to be as effective as DFO in reducing liver iron and maintaining safe serum ferritin levels and normal growth progression.[74,79] In a recent study spanning more than 3 years, DFX significantly and continually decreased cardiac iron overload.[100] There was no significant variation in left ventricular ejection fraction over the study period, which remained within the normal range.

In comparison with patients with TM, patients with SCD have a poorer serum ferritin response during chelation therapy.[101] Possible explanations for this finding include the inadequacy of serum ferritin as a marker of iron burden in SCD, slower dose titration, and compliance issues. In the prospective EPIC (Evaluation of Patients' Iron Chelation with Exjade) trial, after 1 year of treatment serum ferritin levels were significantly decreased in all patients receiving DFX except patients with SCD. However, during the extension study of DFO versus DFX in patients with SCD, those who continued DFX or switched from DFO to DFX significantly decreased their ferritin levels, especially once the average dose was increased to more than 20 mg/kg/d.[102]

In a randomized comparison trial of DFO and DFX in adult and pediatric patients with SCD, a similar reduction of LIC was found in the 2 treatment groups.[75]

Concomitant use with nonsteroidal anti-inflammatory drugs that are often used for pain in SCD, as well as with corticosteroids, oral bisphosphonates, or anticoagulants, should be avoided if possible because of the risk of ulceration and bleeding in the gastrointestinal tract.

Kidney involvement is a well-known complication of SCD. Because of its toxicity profile, concerns about the renal safety of DFX in patients with SCD have been raised. The drug seems to mildly influence renal hemodynamics in the short term (8 weeks), with a decrease in renal plasma flow, leading to a decrease in glomerular filtration rate, which is reversible after drug discontinuation.[103] In a 5-year study by Vichinsky and colleagues,[102] creatinine clearance remained within normal range in patients with SCD.

In the initial study of MRI in children, no patient under the age of 9.5 years was found to have cardiac iron.[105] Subsequently, a study from Brazil reported cardiac iron to be present in 4 of 23 chronically transfused patients ranging in age from 7 to 18 years (**Box 6**), 3 of which were boys under the age of 10 who had received irregular or late chelation therapy.[106] The authors demonstrated by MRI the presence of cardiac iron (T2*<20) and moderate-to-severe liver siderosis in 4 of 35 children under the age of 10.[107,108]

Table 1
Characteristics of the 3 commercially available iron chelators

	Deferoxamine[54]	Deferiprone[55]	Deferasirox[56]
US Food and Drug Administration (FDA) approval	1982 (500 mg vial); 2000 (2 g vial)	2011	2005
European Medicines Agency (EMEA) approval	—	1999	2006
Brands and trademarks	Desferal, Novartis Generic products by several manufacturers (Bedford, Fresnius Kabi USA, Hospira, Watson Labs)	Ferriprox, Apotex Inc Kelfer, Cipla Ltd, India	Exjade, Novartis
Molecular structure	N-[5-[3-[(5-aminopentyl) hydroxycarbamoyl] propionamido]pentyl]-3[[5-(N-hydroxyacetamido)pentyl] carbamoyl] propionohydroxamic acid monomethanesulfonate	3-hydroxy-1,2-dimethylpyridin-4-one	4-[3,5-Bis(2-hydroxyphenyl)-1H-1,2,4-triazol-1-yl] benzoic acid

Indications	Acute iron intoxication Chronic iron overload secondary to transfusion-dependent anemias	Chronic iron overload in patients with TM when deferoxamine (DFO) is contraindicated or inadequate	FDA: Transfusional hemosiderosis in patients 2 y of age and older Chronic iron overload in NTD TM with LIC $\geq$5 mg/g dry weight and serum ferritin >300 μg/L EMEA: Chronic transfusional hemosiderosis in patients with TM 6 y of age and older Treatment of chronic transfusional iron overload when DFO is contraindicated or inadequate in patients with TM aged 2 to 5 y; in TM patients with iron overload due to infrequent blood transfusions aged 2 y and older; in patients with other anemias aged 2 y and older Chronic iron overload in patients with non transfusion dependent thalassemia syndromes aged 10 y and older when DFO is contraindicated or inadequate
Age	None	Limited data <6 y of age	>2 y of age
Dose	20–50 mg/kg/d SC over 8–24 h through a portable pump	75–99 mg/kg/d in 3 daily doses	10–40 mg/kg/d in single dose, according to transfusional iron intake
Available formulations	500 mg and 2 g vials of DFO mesylate USP in sterile, lyophilized form	500 mg and 1 g film-coated tablets 100 mg/mL oral solution	125 mg, 250 mg, 500 mg tablets for oral suspension
Metabolism	Plasma enzymes	Liver glucuronidation	Uridil glucuronosyltransferase enzymes
Iron excretion	Mainly urine; in some patients fecal excretion up to 40%	Mainly urine	Mainly feces

Table 2
Most common and severe adverse effects of iron chelators

Drug	Adverse Effects	Management	Recommendations
DFO	Local side effects at the subcutaneous injection site	Verify correct positioning of needle; hydrocortisone infused with DFO	Adjust dose to serum ferritin levels
	Stunted growth and bone changes (eg, metaphyseal dysplasia)[57,58]	Reduce dose or change chelator	Monitor weight, height, and growth velocity
	Hypersensitivity reactions and systemic allergic reactions	Change treatment drug or desensitization[59,60]	every 3 mo in children
	High-frequency sensorineural hearing loss[61,62]	Rare if dosage guidelines followed and dose adjusted when ferritin declines; if abnormal tests or symptoms, discontinue treatment	Visual acuity tests, slit-lamp examination, and fundoscopy annually
	Visual disturbance[63,64]		Audiometry annually
	Increased serum creatinine, acute renal failure, and renal tubular disorders[65,66]	Reduce dose or discontinue treatment	Monitor renal function periodically
	Increased susceptibility to *Yersinia enterocolitica* and pseudotuberculosis[67] and *Klebsiella pneumoniae* infections[68]	Discontinue treatment if suspected signs and symptoms. Initiate antibiotic therapy	
DFP	Nausea, abdominal pain, vomiting, diarrhea	Usually transient without need to modify treatment; otherwise reduce dose and then increase gradually; as an alternative, switch to oral solution	Weekly neutrophil count
			Monitor hepatic and renal functions periodically
	Neutropenia (neutrophils 0.5–1.5 × 10^9/L)[69]	Discontinue DFP and repeat neutrophil count daily until normalization; rechallenge with caution	Monitor weight and body mass index
	Agranulocytosis (neutrophils <0.5 × 10^9/L on 2 consecutive tests)[69]	Immediately discontinue DFP; if signs/symptoms of infection, perform cultures and begin antibiotic treatment; granulocyte colony stimulating factor may be indicated	Avoid use with other neutropenia-inducing drugs
	Increased liver enzymes[69,70]	Usually asymptomatic and transient without need to modify treatment but may require lowering dose and gradually raising again	
	Increased appetite	Dietary measures	
	Zinc deficiency[71]	Oral zinc supplementation	
	Arthralgia and arthropathy[72,73]	Mild arthralgia is usually transient; if more severe disease, reduce dose or discontinue treatment	
	Neurologic disorders	Described in children taking long-term 2.5 times maximum recommended dose, often in absence of systemic iron overload; discontinue DFP	

(continued on next page)

Table 2
(continued)

Drug	Adverse Effects	Management	Recommendations
DFX	Nausea, vomiting, and abdominal pain[74,75]	Usually transient; if needed reduce dose or discontinue treatment	Monitor serum creatinine, creatinine clearance, and/ or plasma cystatin C twice before initiation, weekly in the first month after initiation, or modification of therapy and then monthly Monthly urinalysis for proteinuria monthly Monitor renal tubular function as needed Monitor serum transaminases, bilirubin, and alkaline phosphatase before initiation of treatment, every 2 wk during the first month, and then monthly Auditory and ophthalmic testing annually
	Diarrhea (may be due to coexistent lactose intolerance)	Consider administration with lactase-containing products	
	Rash	Discontinue DFX; reintroduce at a lower dose after resolution (if necessary add short course of corticosteroids)	
	Increased serum creatinine, proteinuria, acute renal failure, renal tubulopathy, Fanconi syndrome[74,76–78]	Reduce dose by 10 mg/kg if increase in serum creatinine by >33% above pretreatment average and if estimated creatinine clearance decreases below the lower limit of normal at 2 consecutive visits or if abnormalities of tubular markers; if no improvement, change chelator. For more severe changes, consider discontinuing DFX	
	Increased liver enzymes, hepatic failure[74,79]	If persistent and progressive increase in serum transaminases, interrupt treatment; once normalized, cautious reinitiation at a lower dose	
	Upper gastrointestinal ulceration and hemorrhage	Observe carefully in patients in treatment with other potentially ulcerogenic drugs; discontinue treatment if signs or symptoms	
	Auditory (decreased hearing) and ocular (lens opacities) disturbances	Reduce dose or discontinue treatment	
	Cytopenias[80]	Discontinue treatment	

New Chelators

The results of a multicenter phase 2 study designed to assess safety, tolerability, and pharmacodynamics of FBS0701, a novel oral chelator, showed a modest decrease in LIC at the higher dose. The safety and tolerability profile at therapeutic doses seemed to compare favorably to other oral chelators.[109] Further studies are currently underway.

Combination Therapy

Combination therapy, consisting of the use of 2 chelators on the same day, induces negative iron balance in patients with severe iron overload. Balance studies have

---

Box 2
Parameters to be considered when choosing a chelator

- Severity of iron overload
- Transfusional iron intake
- Effectiveness
- Toxicity
- Chelator availability
- Route of administration
- Adherence
- Patient's preference
- Cost

Box 3
Deferoxamine

- DFO was the first chelating agent introduced in clinical practice.
- It has a large molecular weight and a short plasma half-life.
- It is not efficiently absorbed from the gut and negative balance is rarely obtained after intramuscular injection; therefore, it is now usually administered subcutaneously, by means of a portable, battery-operated pump or an elastomeric balloon, over 8–12 hours at night.
- DFO as a continuous intravenous infusion is very effective in reversing severe cardiac iron overload and iron-induced congestive heart failure.
- It efficiently binds non-transferrin-bound iron, preventing free radical formation and lipid peroxidation.[81]
- In patients with SCD, the safety and efficacy of high-dose intravenous DFO were demonstrated by liver biopsy.[82]

Box 4
Deferiprone

- DFP was the first oral chelator to be introduced in clinical practice.
- It is particularly effective in clearing iron from the heart.
- The use in children is limited by the scarcity of data in this population of patients.
- Increasing the dose to 100 mg/kg/d increases the iron excretion without increasing the adverse effects.[87]
- There are limited data on the use of DFP in SCD.[88]

Box 5
Deferasirox

- DFX is as effective as DFO, when administered at the dose of 20 and 30 mg/kg. The rate of transfusional iron intake, however, strongly influences the effectiveness of DFX.
- For most patients with transfusional iron intake averaging less than 0.3 mg/kg/d, a dose of 20 mg/kg of DFX is effective in reducing LIC, whereas an iron intake of greater than 0.5 mg/kg/d requires doses greater than 30 mg/kg/d.[53]
- Doses of up to 40 mg/kg/d are approved for use.

Box 6
Chelation

When to start chelation?[104]

- After receiving 10–12 transfusions
- When the serum ferritin level is consistently greater than 1000 μg/L

What drug should be used?[104]

- Children <2 years old should be started on *subcutaneous DFO infusions* (20–30 mg/kg/5–6 times per week)
- In children age greater than 2 years, *DFX* can be used as first-line chelation
- In children aged greater than 6 years, *DFP liquid formulation* can also be used as a second-line therapy

When to check for organ iron overload in children?[27]

- MRI starting from 6–7 years of age or earlier when poor adherence to chelation is suspected or when blood consumption is increased.

---

shown an additive effect of combination therapy, probably because the 2 drugs access different pools of iron. It has been suggested that DFP, which is able to pass through membranes, could "shuttle" tissue iron to DFO in the bloodstream and then be reused.[110]

Extensive long-term experience has shown that combined chelation with DFP and DFO rapidly reduces liver iron, serum ferritin, and myocardial siderosis, improves cardiac function,[111–113] prevents and reverses endocrine complications, reduces cardiac mortality, and improves survival.[37,114–116] Results of multivariable analysis in the Cypriot TM population demonstrated a 7.4-fold improvement in survival for each year on combination therapy.[117] A recent consensus statement on the treatment of cardiac complications of TM concluded that combined DFP and DFO are superior to DFO alone.[40]

New Combinations

Recently, other combinations of chelators have been tried, all with satisfactory results. A 34-day metabolic iron balance study in 6 patients compared the relative effectiveness of DFX (30 mg/kg/d) and DFO (40 mg/kg/d) alone and in combination. Daily use of both drugs had a synergistic effect in 2 patients and an additive effect in 3 other patients (**Fig. 5**). The authors concluded that supplementing the daily use of DFX with 2 to 3 days of DFO therapy would place all patients in net negative iron balance.[118]

Two reports of simultaneous daily administration of the iron chelators DFX and DFO and of the 2 oral chelators DFX and DFP demonstrated beneficial effects on iron overload of the heart and liver.[119,120] In another study combining the 2 oral chelators DFP and DFX, Berdoukas and colleagues[121] obtained rapid improvement in cardiac iron in 3 patients with severe cardiac iron overload (T2*<6 ms), accompanied by increased ejection fraction in one of the patients who presented with ventricular dysfunction.

Alternating Therapy

When different chelators are given on different days, the chelating regime is called alternating. It should decrease the side effects of chelators and improve compliance. Aydinok and coworkers alternated DFP 4 days a week and DFO on weekends in a

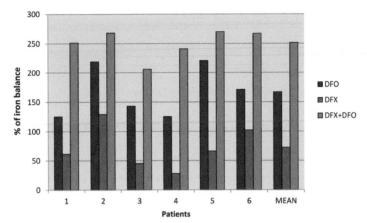

Fig. 5. Iron balance in response to DFO alone (40 mg/kg/d), DFX alone (30 mg/kg/d), and the combination of the 2.

small group of schoolchildren, and they observed an improvement in compliance and a nonsignificant decrease in serum ferritin.[122]

In another multi-institutional study, alternating DFO and DFP gave satisfactory efficacy, but side effects were not reduced much in comparison with either drug alone.[123] A 5-year study, in which 213 patients were randomized to receive alternating DFP-DFO or DFP alone, demonstrated a significantly greater decrease in serum ferritin concentration in the alternating group.[124]

In one report, alternating DFP and DFX allowed treatment of 2 patients who had developed severe side effects with these chelators as well as DFO.[125]

Can Ferritin Be Too Low?

New and intensive therapies have brought to light a new problem. Many physicians wonder whether successful chelation should be discontinued when the ferritin level drops to a particular level, such as 500 ng/mL. Although there are no definitive data answering this question, the authors' large study on survival and complications showed that the risk of death continued to decrease significantly with decreasing ferritin levels down to a value of 1000 ng/mL.[36] Too few patients with lower ferritin levels were available for evaluation. A prospective study of pediatric and adult patients with β-thalassemia treated with DFX for up to 5 years did not show an adverse effect on growth or adolescent sexual development when serum ferritin levels of ~1000 ng/mL were obtained and maintained.[74] Farmaki and colleagues[114] reported reversal of some endocrine complications when normal levels of ferritin were obtained and maintained.

At very low levels of ferritin, dose reduction can be considered, but chelation should never be stopped in transfusion-dependent patients because of the continuing influx of iron and the need to keep labile plasma iron and its potential oxidative damage under control.

Compliance

The role of adherence to therapy is of paramount importance for the success of a chelation regimen. Although the introduction of oral chelators has improved compliance, the effect has not been as great as one might have expected (**Table 3**). Involvement of

Table 3
Reported compliance to iron chelation treatment

Drug	Disease	Adherence	Reference
DFO	TM	59%–78%	[126]
DFP	TM	79%–96%	[126]
DFX	SCD	71% reported by patients 43% documented with pill counts	[127]

patients in the decisions regarding treatment is important and can be obtained in different ways. For example, thorough reviews of MRI results or serial ferritin levels are good methods to develop a therapeutic alliance between caregivers and patients.

The authors have prepared a short video that is shown to young patients while the doctor or the nurse explains how to take the chelators and the importance of adherence to therapy (Video 1).

Chelation After Bone Marrow Transplantation

After allogeneic stem cell transplantation, the iron accumulated during the years of transfusion remains a cause of morbidity. Phlebotomy is the most effective and rapid way to remove iron. However, some patients, especially those who receive their stem cells from a donor with a thalassemia trait, may not achieve a hemoglobin level high enough to allow blood removal, and therefore, they need chelation therapy at least for a few months. Both DFO and DFX have been used successfully in this setting.[128–131]

Costs

The costs of chelation therapy differ from drug to drug and from country to country. The prices in 3 countries are reported in **Table 4**. Several studies have evaluated the cost-effectiveness of different chelators in terms of quality of life. Most suggest an advantage of oral chelators versus DFO.[132]

Two studies comparing the 3 chelators favored DFP over the other 2 because of better cost-effectiveness.[95,133]

Availability of Chelation

Hemoglobinopathies are found worldwide and are particularly common in countries with limited resources. Because both transfusion and chelation are expensive therapies, many children die without the benefit of treatment. **Table 5** presents data on TM collected by Modell and Darlison.[134]

Table 4
Daily costs of chelation treatment with 3 different drugs in 3 countries (calculated for a patient of 70 kg)

Drug	Italy Cost per day (€)	UK Cost per day (£)	USA Cost per day ($)
DFP	19.45	18.66	307.35
DFO	12.10–20.61	13.68	115–117 (2 g)
DFX	72.8–109.2	60.48	341.48

Table 5
Estimated reach of treatment for β-thalassemia in each World Health Organization (WHO) region[a]

WHO Region	Estimated Annual Birth β-Thalassemias Transfusion Dependent	Transfusion		Adequate Iron Chelation %	Inadequate or No Iron Chelation	
		% of Transfusion-dependent Patients Transfused	Annual Deaths Because Not Transfused		No. of Patients	Annual Deaths due to Iron Overload
African	1278	2.7	1243	—	—	—
American	255	52.4	121	58	1146	57
Eastern Mediterranean	9053	17.8	7443	27	28,882	1444
European	920	15.5	780	91	1476	74
Southeast Asian	9983	9.6	9021	19	28,879	1444
Western Pacific	4022	2.7	3914	44	1946	97
World	25,511	11.7	22,522	39	59,764	2988

[a] All figures are minimum estimates.

SUMMARY

The availability of iron chelation has changed the prognosis for patients with TM, first with the introduction of DFO and, later, with the oral chelators. Further significant improvement can be expected in the future as a consequence of the availability of new chelators and of better combined use of the present ones. Also, MRI techniques for measuring iron overload in the different organs will allow earlier diagnosis and tailored therapy. The degree to which these benefits will accrue in other disorders in which patients receive regular transfusions will depend on the severity of iron-induced organ damage and the impact of the underlying disease on survival.

Most children with TM and SCD are born in low-income countries, where there is an urgent need for correct treatment combined with prevention programs. Most transfused patients with TM will die from iron overload unless an inexpensive oral iron chelator becomes available.[134]

Patients with SCD often die undiagnosed in infancy, usually from malaria or infections. Now, however, improved access to health care is leading to increased survival.[134] As patients live longer and as transfusion therapy becomes more widely available, the need for chelation therapy will almost certainly increase.

SUPPLEMENTARY DATA

Supplementary data related to this article can be found online at http://dx.doi.org/10.1016/j.hoc.2014.04.004.

REFERENCES

1. Quinn CT, Rogers ZR, Buchanan GR. Survival of children with sickle cell disease. Blood 2004;103(11):4023–7. http://dx.doi.org/10.1182/blood-2003-11-3758.
2. Quinn CT, Rogers ZR, McCavit TL, et al. Improved survival of children and adolescents with sickle cell disease. Blood 2010;115(17):3447–52. http://dx.doi.org/10.1182/blood-2009-07-233700.

3. Lee A, Thomas P, Cupidore L, et al. Improved survival in homozygous sickle cell disease: lessons from a cohort study. BMJ 1995;311(7020):1600–2. Available at: http://www.pubmedcentral.nih.gov/articlerender.fcgi?artid=2551498&tool=pmcentrez&rendertype=abstract. Accessed July 11, 2012.
4. Serjeant GR, Serjeant BE, Mason KP, et al. The changing face of homozygous sickle cell disease: 102 patients over 60 years. Int J Lab Hematol 2009;31(6):585–96. http://dx.doi.org/10.1111/j.1751-553X.2008.01089.x.
5. Vichinsky EP. Current issues with blood transfusions in sickle cell disease. Semin Hematol 2001;38(1 Suppl 1):14–22. Available at: http://www.ncbi.nlm.nih.gov/pubmed/11206956. Accessed September 22, 2013.
6. Wahl S, Quirolo KC. Current issues in blood transfusion for sickle cell disease. Curr Opin Pediatr 2009;21(1):15–21. http://dx.doi.org/10.1097/MOP.0b013e328321882e.
7. Uchida K, Rackoff WR, Ohene-Frempong K, et al. Effect of erythrocytapheresis on arterial oxygen saturation and hemoglobin oxygen affinity in patients with sickle cell disease. Am J Hematol 1998;59(1):5–8. Available at: http://www.ncbi.nlm.nih.gov/pubmed/9723569. Accessed July 12, 2012.
8. Switzer JA, Hess DC, Nichols FT, et al. Pathophysiology and treatment of stroke in sickle-cell disease: present and future. Lancet Neurol 2006;5(6):501–12. http://dx.doi.org/10.1016/S1474-4422(06)70469-0.
9. Dunbar LN, Coleman Brown L, Rivera DR, et al. Transfusion practices in the management of sickle cell disease: a survey of Florida hematologists/oncologists. ISRN Hematol 2012;2012:524513. http://dx.doi.org/10.5402/2012/524513.
10. Hirst C, Williamson L. Preoperative blood transfusions for sickle cell disease [review]. Cochrane Database Syst Rev 2012;(1):CD003149.
11. Vichinsky EP, Haberkern CM, Neumayr L, et al. A comparison of conservative and aggressive transfusion regimens in the perioperative management of sickle cell disease. The Preoperative Transfusion in Sickle Cell Disease Study Group. N Engl J Med 1995;333(4):206–13. http://dx.doi.org/10.1056/NEJM19950727333 30402.
12. Brousse V, Elie C, Benkerrou M, et al. Acute splenic sequestration crisis in sickle cell disease: cohort study of 190 paediatric patients. Br J Haematol 2012; 156(5):643–8. http://dx.doi.org/10.1111/j.1365-2141.2011.08999.x.
13. Al-Salem AH. Splenic complications of sickle cell anemia and the role of splenectomy. ISRN Hematol 2011;2011:864257. http://dx.doi.org/10.5402/2011/864257.
14. Booth C, Inusa B, Obaro SK. Infection in sickle cell disease: a review. Int J Infect Dis 2010;14(1):e2–12. http://dx.doi.org/10.1016/j.ijid.2009.03.010.
15. Laurie GA. Acute chest syndrome in sickle cell disease. Intern Med J 2010; 40(5):372–6. http://dx.doi.org/10.1111/j.1445-5994.2010.02129.x.
16. Miller AC, Gladwin MT. Pulmonary complications of sickle cell disease. Am J Respir Crit Care Med 2012;185(11):1154–65. http://dx.doi.org/10.1164/rccm. 201111-2082CI.
17. Islam MS, Anoop P. Current concepts in the management of stroke in children with sickle cell disease. Childs Nerv Syst 2011;27(7):1037–43. http://dx.doi.org/10.1007/s00381-011-1394-0.
18. Webb J, Kwiatkowski JL. Stroke in patients with sickle cell disease. Expert Rev Hematol 2013;6(3):301–16. http://dx.doi.org/10.1586/ehm.13.25.
19. Hiran S. Multiorgan dysfunction syndrome in sickle cell disease. J Assoc Physicians India 2005;53:19–22. Available at: http://www.ncbi.nlm.nih.gov/pubmed/15857006. Accessed September 26, 2013.
20. Adams R, McKie V, Hsu L, et al. Prevention of a first stroke by transfusions in children with sickle cell anemia and abnormal results on transcranial Doppler

ultrasonography. N Engl J Med 1998;339:5–11. Available at: http://www.nejm.org/doi/full/10.1056/NEJM199807023390102. Accessed July 10, 2012.

21. Adams RJ, Brambilla D. Discontinuing prophylactic transfusions used to prevent stroke in sickle cell disease. N Engl J Med 2005;353(26):2769–78. http://dx.doi.org/10.1056/NEJMoa050460.

22. Miller ST, Wright E, Abboud M, et al. Impact of chronic transfusion on incidence of pain and acute chest syndrome during the Stroke Prevention Trial (STOP) in sickle-cell anemia. J Pediatr 2001;139(6):785–9. http://dx.doi.org/10.1067/mpd.2001.119593.

23. Kalff A, Dowsing C, Grigg A. The impact of a regular erythrocytapheresis programme on the acute and chronic complications of sickle cell disease in adults. Br J Haematol 2010;149(5):768–74. http://dx.doi.org/10.1111/j.1365-2141.2010.08150.x.

24. Hankins J, Jeng M, Harris S, et al. Chronic transfusion therapy for children with sickle cell disease and recurrent acute chest syndrome. J Pediatr Hematol Oncol 2005;27(3):158–61. Available at: http://www.ncbi.nlm.nih.gov/pubmed/15750449. Accessed September 28, 2013.

25. Cho G, Ir H. Regular long-term red blood cell transfusions for managing chronic chest complications in sickle cell disease [review]. Cochrane Database Syst Rev 2011;(9):CD008360.

26. Singer ST, Quirolo K, Nishi K, et al. Erythrocytapheresis for chronically transfused children with sickle cell disease: an effective method for maintaining a low hemoglobin S level and reducing iron overload. J Clin Apheresis 1999;14(3):122–5. Available at: http://www.ncbi.nlm.nih.gov/pubmed/10540366. Accessed December 7, 2013.

27. Cappellini MD, Cohen AR, Eleftheriou A. Guidelines for the clinical management of thalassemia. 2nd edition. Nicosia (Cyprus): Thalassaemia International Federation; 2008.

28. Bracey AW, Klein HG, Chambers S, et al. Ex vivo selective isolation of young red blood cells using the IBM-2991 cell washer. Blood 1983;61(6):1068–71. Available at: http://www.ncbi.nlm.nih.gov/pubmed/6839016. Accessed December 17, 2013.

29. Esposito BP, Breuer W, Sirankapracha P, et al. Labile plasma iron in iron overload: redox activity and susceptibility to chelation. Blood 2003;102(7):2670–7. http://dx.doi.org/10.1182/blood-2003-03-0807.

30. Cartwright GE, Edwards CQ, Kravitz K, et al. Hereditary hemochromatosis. Phenotypic expression of the disease. N Engl J Med 1979;301(4):175–9. http://dx.doi.org/10.1056/NEJM197907263010402.

31. King L, Reid M, Forrester TE. Iron deficiency anaemia in Jamaican children, aged 1-5 years, with sickle cell disease. West Indian Med J 2005;54(5):292–6. Available at: http://www.ncbi.nlm.nih.gov/pubmed/16459510. Accessed July 14, 2012.

32. Walter PB, Harmatz P, Vichinsky E. Iron metabolism and iron chelation in sickle cell disease. Acta Haematol 2009;122(2–3):174–83. http://dx.doi.org/10.1159/000243802.

33. Walter PB, Fung EB, Killilea DW, et al. Oxidative stress and inflammation in iron-overloaded patients with beta-thalassaemia or sickle cell disease. Br J Haematol 2006;135(2):254–63. http://dx.doi.org/10.1111/j.1365-2141.2006.06277.x.

34. Vichinsky E, Butensky E, Fung E. Comparison of organ dysfunction in transfused patients with SCD or beta thalassemia. Am J Hematol 2005;80:70–4. Available at: http://onlinelibrary.wiley.com/doi/10.1002/ajh.20402/abstract. Accessed July 10, 2012.

35. Marsella M, Borgna-Pignatti C, Meloni A, et al. Cardiac iron and cardiac disease in males and females with transfusion-dependent thalassemia major: a T2*

magnetic resonance imaging study. Haematologica 2011;96(4):515–20. http://dx.doi.org/10.3324/haematol.2010.025510.

36. Borgna-Pignatti C, Rugolotto S, De Stefano P, et al. Survival and complications in patients with thalassemia major treated with transfusion and deferoxamine. Haematologica 2004;89(10):1187–93.

37. Telfer P, Coen PG, Christou S, et al. Survival of medically treated thalassemia patients in Cyprus. Trends and risk factors over the period 1980-2004. Haematologica 2006;91(9):1187–92.

38. Mokhtar GM, Gadallah M, El Sherif NH, et al. Morbidities and mortality in transfusion-dependent beta-thalassemia patients (single-center experience). Pediatr Hematol Oncol 2013;30(2):93–103. http://dx.doi.org/10.3109/08880018.2012.752054.

39. Au WY, Lee V, Lau CW, et al. A synopsis of current care of thalassaemia major patients in Hong Kong. Hong Kong Med J 2011;17(4):261–6. Available at: http://www.ncbi.nlm.nih.gov/pubmed/21813892. Accessed April 10, 2014.

40. Pennell DJ, Udelson JE, Arai AE, et al. Cardiovascular function and treatment in β-thalassemia major: a consensus statement from the American Heart Association. Circulation 2013;128(3):281–308. http://dx.doi.org/10.1161/CIR.0b013e31829b2be6.

41. Inati A, Musallam KM, Wood JC, et al. Absence of cardiac siderosis by MRI T2* despite transfusion burden, hepatic and serum iron overload in Lebanese patients with sickle cell disease. Eur J Haematol 2009;83(6):565–71. http://dx.doi.org/10.1111/j.1600-0609.2009.01345.x.

42. Voskaridou E, Douskou M, Terpos E, et al. Magnetic resonance imaging in the evaluation of iron overload in patients with beta thalassaemia and sickle cell disease. Br J Haematol 2004;126(5):736–42. http://dx.doi.org/10.1111/j.1365-2141.2004.05104.x.

43. Wood JC, Tyszka JM, Carson S, et al. Myocardial iron loading in transfusion-dependent thalassemia and sickle cell disease. Blood 2004;103(5):1934–6. http://dx.doi.org/10.1182/blood-2003-06-1919.

44. Angelucci E, Muretto P, Nicolucci A, et al. Effects of iron overload and hepatitis C virus positivity in determining progression of liver fibrosis in thalassemia following bone marrow transplantation. Blood 2002;100(1):17–21.

45. Borgna-Pignatti C, Cappellini MD, De Stefano P, et al. Cardiac morbidity and mortality in deferoxamine- or deferiprone-treated patients with thalassemia major. Blood 2006;107(9):3733–7. http://dx.doi.org/10.1182/blood-2005-07-2933.

46. Perifanis V, Tziomalos K, Tsatra I, et al. Prevalence and severity of liver disease in patients with b thalassemia major. A single-institution fifteen-year experience. Haematologica 2005;90(8):1136–8. Available at: http://www.ncbi.nlm.nih.gov/pubmed/16079116. Accessed December 10, 2013.

47. Anderson LJ, Holden S, Davis B, et al. Cardiovascular T2-star (T2*) magnetic resonance for the early diagnosis of myocardial iron overload. Eur Heart J 2001;22(23):2171–9.

48. Hankins J, Smeltzer M. Patterns of liver iron accumulation in patients with sickle cell disease and thalassemia with iron overload. Eur J 2010;85(1):51–7. http://dx.doi.org/10.1111/j.1600-0609.2010.01449.x.Patterns.

49. Hassan M, Hasan S, Giday S, et al. Hepatitis C virus in sickle cell disease. J Natl Med Assoc 2003;95(10):939–42. Available at: http://www.pubmedcentral.nih.gov/articlerender.fcgi?artid=2594496&tool=pmcentrez&rendertype=abstract. Accessed November 26, 2013.

50. Namasopo S, Ndugwa C, Tumwine J. Hepatitis C and blood transfusion among children attending the Sickle Cell Clinic at Mulago Hospital, Uganda. Afr Health Sci 2013;13(2):255–60. http://dx.doi.org/10.4314/ahs.v13i2.8.
51. Ejiofor OS, Ibe BC, Emodi IJ, et al. The role of blood transfusion on the prevalence of hepatitis C virus antibodies in children with sickle cell anaemia in Enugu, South East Nigeria. Niger J Clin Pract 2009;12(4):355–8. Available at: http://www.ncbi.nlm.nih.gov/pubmed/20329670. Accessed November 26, 2013.
52. Fung EB, Harmatz PR, Lee PD, et al. Increased prevalence of iron-overload associated endocrinopathy in thalassaemia versus sickle-cell disease. Br J Haematol 2006;135(4):574–82. http://dx.doi.org/10.1111/j.1365-2141.2006.06332.x.
53. Cohen AR, Glimm E, Porter JB. Effect of transfusional iron intake on response to chelation therapy in beta-thalassemia major. Blood 2008;111(2):583–7. http://dx.doi.org/10.1182/blood-2007-08-109306.
54. Desferal summary of product characteristics. 3–12. Available at: http://www.pharma.us.novartis.com/product/pi/pdf/desferal.pdf.
55. Ferriprox summary of product characteristics. 1–56. Available at: http://www.ema.europa.eu/docs/en_GB/document_library/EPAR_-_Product_Information/human/000236/WC500022050.pdf.
56. Exjade summary of product characteristics. 1–73. Available at: http://www.ema.europa.eu/docs/en_GB/document_library/EPAR_-_Product_Information/human/000670/WC500033925.pdf.
57. Olivieri NF, Koren G, Harris J, et al. Growth failure and bony changes induced by deferoxamine. Am J Pediatr Hematol Oncol 1992;14(1):48–56.
58. De Virgiliis S, Congia M, Frau F, et al. Deferoxamine-induced growth retardation in patients with thalassemia major. J Pediatr 1988;113(4):661–9.
59. Cianciulli P, Sorrentino F, Maffei L, et al. Continuous low-dose subcutaneous desferrioxamine (DFO) to prevent allergic manifestations in patients with iron overload. Ann Hematol 1996;73(6):279–81.
60. Bousquet J, Navarro M, Robert G, et al. Rapid desensitisation for desferrioxamine anaphylactoid reaction. Lancet 1983;2(8354):859–60.
61. Olivieri NF, Buncic JR, Chew E, et al. Visual and auditory neurotoxicity in patients receiving subcutaneous deferoxamine infusions. N Engl J Med 1986;314(14):869–73. http://dx.doi.org/10.1056/NEJM198604033141402.
62. Gallant T, Boyden MH, Gallant LA, et al. Serial studies of auditory neurotoxicity in patients receiving deferoxamine therapy. Am J Med 1987;83(6):1085–90.
63. Davies S, Hungerford JL, Arden GB, et al. Ocular toxicity of high-dose intravenous desferrioxamine. Lancet 1983;322(8343):181–4. http://dx.doi.org/10.1016/S0140-6736(83)90170-8.
64. Borgna-Pignatti C, De Stefano P, Broglia AM. Visual loss in patient on high-dose subcutaneous desferrioxamine. Lancet 1984;1(8378):681.
65. Koren G, Bentur Y, Strong D, et al. Acute changes in renal function associated with deferoxamine therapy. Am J Dis Child 1989;143(9):1077–80.
66. Koren G, Kochavi-Atiya Y, Bentur Y, et al. The effects of subcutaneous deferoxamine administration on renal function in thalassemia major. Int J Hematol 1991;54(5):371–5.
67. Robins-Browne RM, Prpic JK, Stuart SJ. Yersiniae and iron. A study in host-parasite relationships. Contrib Microbiol Immunol 1987;9:254–8.
68. Chan GC, Chan S, Ho PL, et al. Effects of chelators (deferoxamine, deferiprone and deferasirox) on the growth of Klebsiella pneumoniae and Aeromonas hydrophila isolated from transfusion-dependent thalassemia patients. Hemoglobin 2009;33(5):352–60. http://dx.doi.org/10.3109/03630260903211888.

69. Cohen AR, Galanello R, Piga A, et al. Safety and effectiveness of long-term therapy with the oral iron chelator deferiprone. Blood 2003;102(5):1583–7. http://dx.doi.org/10.1182/blood-2002-10-3280.
70. al-Refaie FN, Hershko C, Hoffbrand AV, et al. Results of long-term deferiprone (L1) therapy: a report by the International Study Group on Oral Iron Chelators. Br J Haematol 1995;91(1):224–9. Available at: http://www.ncbi.nlm.nih.gov/pubmed/7577638. Accessed November 28, 2013.
71. al-Refaie FN, Wonke B, Wickens DG, et al. Zinc concentration in patients with iron overload receiving oral iron chelator 1,2-dimethyl-3-hydroxypyrid-4-one or desferrioxamine. J Clin Pathol 1994;47(7):657–60.
72. Berkovitch M, Laxer RM, Inman R, et al. Arthropathy in thalassaemia patients receiving deferiprone. Lancet 1994;343(8911):1471–2. Available at: http://www.ncbi.nlm.nih.gov/pubmed/7911181. Accessed November 28, 2013.
73. Chand G, Chowdhury V, Manchanda A, et al. Deferiprone-induced arthropathy in thalassemia: MRI findings in a case. Indian J Radiol Imaging 2009;19(2):155–7. http://dx.doi.org/10.4103/0971-3026.50839.
74. Cappellini MD, Bejaoui M, Agaoglu L, et al. Iron chelation with deferasirox in adult and pediatric patients with thalassemia major: efficacy and safety during 5 years' follow-up. Blood 2011;118(4):884–93. http://dx.doi.org/10.1182/blood-2010-11-316646.
75. Vichinsky E, Onyekwere O, Porter J, et al. A randomised comparison of deferasirox versus deferoxamine for the treatment of transfusional iron overload in sickle cell disease. Br J Haematol 2007;136(3):501–8. http://dx.doi.org/10.1111/j.1365-2141.2006.06455.x.
76. Rafat C, Fakhouri F, Ribeil JA, et al. Fanconi syndrome due to deferasirox. Am J Kidney Dis 2009;54(5):931–4. http://dx.doi.org/10.1053/j.ajkd.2009.03.013.
77. Rheault MN, Bechtel H, Neglia JP, et al. Reversible Fanconi syndrome in a pediatric patient on deferasirox. Pediatr Blood Cancer 2011;56(4):674–6. http://dx.doi.org/10.1002/pbc.22711.
78. Wei HY, Yang CP, Cheng CH, et al. Fanconi syndrome in a patient with β-thalassemia major after using deferasirox for 27 months. Transfusion 2011;51(5):949–54. http://dx.doi.org/10.1111/j.1537-2995.2010.02939.x.
79. Cappellini MD. A phase 3 study of deferasirox (ICL670), a once-daily oral iron chelator, in patients with beta-thalassemia. Blood 2006;107(9):3455–62. http://dx.doi.org/10.1182/blood-2005-08-3430.
80. Grandvuillemin A, Audia S, Leguy-Seguin V, et al. Severe thrombocytopenia and mild leucopenia associated with deferasirox therapy. Therapie 2009;64(6):405–7 [in French].
81. Breuer W, Ronson A, Slotki IN, et al. The assessment of serum nontransferrin-bound iron in chelation therapy and iron supplementation. Blood 2000;95(9):2975–82.
82. Kalpatthi R, Peters B, Kane I, et al. Safety and efficacy of high dose intravenous desferrioxamine for reduction of iron overload in sickle cell disease. Pediatr Blood Cancer 2010;55(7):1338–42. http://dx.doi.org/10.1002/pbc.22660.
83. Anderson LJ, Westwood MA, Holden S, et al. Myocardial iron clearance during reversal of siderotic cardiomyopathy with intravenous desferrioxamine: a prospective study using T2* cardiovascular magnetic resonance. Br J Haematol 2004;127(3):348–55. http://dx.doi.org/10.1111/j.1365-2141.2004.05202.x.
84. Borgna-Pignatti C, Cohen A. Evaluation of a new method of administration of the iron chelating agent deferoxamine. J Pediatr 1997;130(1):86–8.

85. Borgna-Pignatti C, Franchini M, Gandini G, et al. Subcutaneous bolus injection of deferoxamine in adult patients affected by onco-hematologic diseases and iron overload. Haematologica 1998;83(9):788–90.

86. Franchini M, Gandini G, de Gironcoli M, et al. Safety and efficacy of subcutaneous bolus injection of deferoxamine in adult patients with iron overload. Blood 2000;95(9):2776–9.

87. Hoffbrand AV. Oral iron chelation. Semin Hematol 1996;33(1):1–8.

88. Lucania G, Vitrano A, Filosa A, et al. Chelation treatment in sickle-cell-anaemia: much ado about nothing? Br J Haematol 2011;154(5):545–55. http://dx.doi.org/10.1111/j.1365-2141.2011.08769.x.

89. Gomber S, Saxena R, Madan N. Comparative efficacy of desferrioxamine, deferiprone and in combination on iron chelation in thalassemic children. Indian Pediatr 2004;41(1):21–7. Available at: http://www.ncbi.nlm.nih.gov/pubmed/14767084. Accessed December 10, 2013.

90. ElAlfy MS, El Alfy M, Sari TT, et al. The safety, tolerability, and efficacy of a liquid formulation of deferiprone in young children with transfusional iron overload. J Pediatr Hematol Oncol 2010;32(8):601–5. http://dx.doi.org/10.1097/MPH.0b013e3181ec0f13.

91. Makis A, Chaliasos N, Alfantaki S, et al. Chelation therapy with oral solution of deferiprone in transfusional iron-overloaded children with hemoglobinopathies. Anemia 2013;2013:121762. http://dx.doi.org/10.1155/2013/121762.

92. Viprakasit V, Nuchprayoon I, Chuansumrit A, et al. Deferiprone (GPO-L-ONE(®)) monotherapy reduces iron overload in transfusion-dependent thalassemias: 1-year results from a multicenter prospective, single arm, open label, dose escalating phase III pediatric study (GPO-L-ONE; A001) from Thailand. Am J Hematol 2013;88(4):251–60. http://dx.doi.org/10.1002/ajh.23386.

93. Efficacy/Safety Study of Deferiprone Compared to Deferasirox in Paediatric Patients - Full Text View. Available at: http://clinicaltrial.gov/ct2/show/NCT01825512?term=deferiprone&rank=16.

94. Voskaridou E, Douskou M, Terpos E, et al. Deferiprone as an oral iron chelator in sickle cell disease. Ann Hematol 2005;84(7):434–40. http://dx.doi.org/10.1007/s00277-005-1015-7.

95. McLeod C, Fleeman N, Kirkham J, et al. Deferasirox for the treatment of iron overload associated with regular blood transfusions (transfusional haemosiderosis) in patients suffering with chronic anaemia: a systematic review and economic evaluation. Health Technol Assess 2009;13(1):iii–iiv, ix–xi, 1–121. http://dx.doi.org/10.3310/hta13010.

96. Piga A, Gaglioti C, Fogliacco E, et al. Comparative effects of deferiprone and deferoxamine on survival and cardiac disease in patients with thalassemia major: a retrospective analysis. Haematologica 2003;88(5):489–96.

97. Ladis V, Chouliaras G, Berdoukas V, et al. Survival in a large cohort of Greek patients with transfusion-dependent beta thalassaemia and mortality ratios compared to the general population. Eur J Haematol 2011;86(4):332–8. http://dx.doi.org/10.1111/j.1600-0609.2011.01582.x.

98. Pennell DJ, Berdoukas V, Karagiorga M, et al. Randomized controlled trial of deferiprone or deferoxamine in beta-thalassemia major patients with asymptomatic myocardial siderosis. Blood 2006;107(9):3738–44. http://dx.doi.org/10.1182/blood-2005-07-2948.

99. Pepe A, Meloni A, Capra M, et al. Deferasirox, deferiprone and desferrioxamine treatment in thalassemia major patients: cardiac iron and function comparison

determined by quantitative magnetic resonance imaging. Haematologica 2011; 96(1):41–7. http://dx.doi.org/10.3324/haematol.2009.019042.

100. Pennell DJ, Porter JB, Cappellini MD, et al. Deferasirox for up to 3 years leads to continued improvement of myocardial T2* in patients with beta-thalassemia major. Haematologica 2012;97(6):842–8. http://dx.doi.org/10.3324/haematol.2011.049957.

101. Cappellini MD, Porter J, El-Beshlawy A, et al. Tailoring iron chelation by iron intake and serum ferritin: the prospective EPIC study of deferasirox in 1744 patients with transfusion-dependent anemias. Haematologica 2010;95(4):557–66. http://dx.doi.org/10.3324/haematol.2009.014696.

102. Vichinsky E, Bernaudin F, Forni GL, et al. Long-term safety and efficacy of deferasirox (Exjade®) for up to 5 years in transfusional iron-overloaded patients with sickle cell disease. Br J Haematol 2011;154(3):387–97. http://dx.doi.org/10.1111/j.1365-2141.2011.08720.x.

103. Galanello R, Campus S, Origa R. Deferasirox: pharmacokinetics and clinical experience. Expert Opin Drug Metab Toxicol 2012;8(1):123–34. http://dx.doi.org/10.1517/17425255.2012.640674.

104. Angelucci E, Barosi G, Camaschella C, et al. Italian Society of Hematology practice guidelines for the management of iron overload in thalassemia major and related disorders. Haematologica 2008;93(5):741–52. http://dx.doi.org/10.3324/haematol.12413.

105. Wood JC, Origa R, Agus A, et al. Onset of cardiac iron loading in pediatric patients with thalassemia major. Haematologica 2008;93(6):917–20. http://dx.doi.org/10.3324/haematol.12513.

106. Fernandes JL, Fabron A, Verissimo M. Early cardiac iron overload in children with transfusion-dependent anemias. Haematologica 2009;94(12):1776–7. http://dx.doi.org/10.3324/haematol.2009.013193.

107. Borgna-Pignatti C, Meloni A, Guerrini G, et al. Myocardial iron overload in thalassaemia major. How early to check? Br J Haematol 2013. http://dx.doi.org/10.1111/bjh.12643.

108. Berdoukas V, Nord A, Carson S, et al. Tissue iron evaluation in chronically transfused children shows significant levels of iron loading at a very young age. Am J Hematol 2013;88(11):E283–5. http://dx.doi.org/10.1002/ajh.23543.

109. Neufeld EJ, Galanello R, Viprakasit V, et al. A phase 2 study of the safety, tolerability, and pharmacodynamics of FBS0701, a novel oral iron chelator, in transfusional iron overload. Blood 2012;119(14):3263–8. http://dx.doi.org/10.1182/blood-2011-10-386268.

110. Link G, Konijn AM, Breuer W, et al. Exploring the "iron shuttle" hypothesis in chelation therapy: effects of combined deferoxamine and deferiprone treatment in hypertransfused rats with labeled iron stores and in iron-loaded rat heart cells in culture. J Lab Clin Med 2001;138(2):130–8. http://dx.doi.org/10.1067/mlc.2001.116487.

111. Alpendurada F, Smith GC, Carpenter J-P, et al. Effects of combined deferiprone with deferoxamine on right ventricular function in thalassaemia major. J Cardiovasc Magn Reson 2012;14:8. http://dx.doi.org/10.1186/1532-429X-14-8.

112. Tanner MA, Galanello R, Dessi C, et al. A randomized, placebo-controlled, double-blind trial of the effect of combined therapy with deferoxamine and deferiprone on myocardial iron in thalassemia major using cardiovascular magnetic resonance. Circulation 2007;115(14):1876–84. http://dx.doi.org/10.1161/CIRCULATIONAHA.106.648790.

113. Daar S, Pathare AV. Combined therapy with desferrioxamine and deferiprone in beta thalassemia major patients with transfusional iron overload. Ann Hematol 2006;85(5):315–9. http://dx.doi.org/10.1007/s00277-005-0075-z.

114. Farmaki K, Tzoumari I, Pappa C, et al. Normalisation of total body iron load with very intensive combined chelation reverses cardiac and endocrine complications of thalassaemia major. Br J Haematol 2010;148(3):466–75. http://dx.doi.org/10.1111/j.1365-2141.2009.07970.x.

115. Maggio A, Vitrano A, Capra M, et al. Improving survival with deferiprone treatment in patients with thalassemia major: a prospective multicenter randomised clinical trial under the auspices of the Italian Society for Thalassemia and Hemoglobinopathies. Blood Cells Mol Dis 2009;42(3):247–51. http://dx.doi.org/10.1016/j.bcmd.2009.01.002.

116. Lai ME, Grady RW, Vacquer S, et al. Increased survival and reversion of iron-induced cardiac disease in patients with thalassemia major receiving intensive combined chelation therapy as compared to desferoxamine alone. Blood Cells Mol Dis 2010;45(2):136–9. http://dx.doi.org/10.1016/j.bcmd.2010.05.005.

117. Telfer PT, Warburton F, Christou S, et al. Improved survival in thalassemia major patients on switching from desferrioxamine to combined chelation therapy with desferrioxamine and deferiprone. Haematologica 2009;94(12):1777–8. http://dx.doi.org/10.3324/haematol.2009.009118.

118. Grady RW, Galanello R, Randolph RE, et al. Toward optimizing the use of deferasirox: potential benefits of combined use with deferoxamine. Haematologica 2013;98(1):129–35. http://dx.doi.org/10.3324/haematol.2012.070607.

119. Voskaridou E, Komninaka V, Karavas A, et al. Combination therapy of deferasirox and deferoxamine shows significant improvements in markers of iron overload in a patient with β-thalassemia major and severe iron burden. Transfusion 2013. http://dx.doi.org/10.1111/trf.12335.

120. Voskaridou E, Christoulas D, Terpos E. Successful chelation therapy with the combination of deferasirox and deferiprone in a patient with thalassaemia major and persisting severe iron overload after single-agent chelation therapies. Br J Haematol 2011;154(5):654–6. http://dx.doi.org/10.1111/j.1365-2141.2011.08626.x.

121. Berdoukas V, Carson S, Nord A, et al. Combining two orally active iron chelators for thalassemia. Ann Hematol 2010;89(11):1177–8. http://dx.doi.org/10.1007/s00277-010-0933-1.

122. Aydinok Y, Nisli G, Kavakli K, et al. Sequential use of deferiprone and desferrioxamine in primary school children with thalassaemia major in Turkey. Acta Haematol 1999;102(1):17–21.

123. Galanello R, Kattamis A, Piga A, et al. A prospective randomized controlled trial on the safety and efficacy of alternating deferoxamine and deferiprone in the treatment of iron overload in patients with thalassemia. Haematologica 2006; 91(9):1241–3.

124. Pantalone GR, Maggio A, Vitrano A, et al. Sequential alternating deferiprone and deferoxamine treatment compared to deferiprone monotherapy: main findings and clinical follow-up of a large multicenter randomized clinical trial in -thalassemia major patients. Hemoglobin 2011;35(3):206–16. http://dx.doi.org/10.3109/03630269.2011.570674.

125. Balocco M, Carrara P, Pinto V, et al. Daily alternating deferasirox and deferiprone therapy for "hard-to-chelate" beta-thalassemia major patients. Am J Hematol 2010;85(6):460–1. http://dx.doi.org/10.1002/ajh.21711.

126. Delea TE, Edelsberg J, Sofrygin O, et al. Consequences and costs of noncompliance with iron chelation therapy in patients with transfusion-dependent thalassemia: a literature review. Transfusion 2007;47(10):1919–29. http://dx.doi.org/10.1111/j.1537-2995.2007.01416.x.
127. Alvarez O, Rodriguez-Cortes H, Robinson N, et al. Adherence to deferasirox in children and adolescents with sickle cell disease during 1-year of therapy. J Pediatr Hematol Oncol 2009;31(10):739–44. http://dx.doi.org/10.1097/MPH.0b013e3181b53363.
128. Yesilipek MA, Karasu G, Kazik M, et al. Posttransplant oral iron-chelating therapy in patients with beta-thalassemia major. Pediatr Hematol Oncol 2010; 27(5):374–9. http://dx.doi.org/10.3109/08880011003739463.
129. Li CK, Lai DH, Shing MM, et al. Early iron reduction programme for thalassaemia patients after bone marrow transplantation. Bone Marrow Transplant 2000;25(6): 653–6. http://dx.doi.org/10.1038/sj.bmt.1702212.
130. Giardini C, Galimberti M, Lucarelli G, et al. Desferrioxamine therapy accelerates clearance of iron deposits after bone marrow transplantation for thalassaemia. Br J Haematol 1995;89(4):868–73. Available at: http://www.ncbi.nlm.nih.gov/pubmed/7772524. Accessed December 7, 2013.
131. Mariotti E, Angelucci E, Agostini A, et al. Evaluation of cardiac status in iron-loaded thalassaemia patients following bone marrow transplantation: improvement in cardiac function during reduction in body iron burden. Br J Haematol 1998;103(4):916–21. Available at: http://www.ncbi.nlm.nih.gov/pubmed/9886301. Accessed December 7, 2013.
132. Karnon J, Tolley K, Vieira J, et al. Lifetime cost-utility analyses of deferasirox in beta-thalassaemia patients with chronic iron overload: a UK perspective. Clin Drug Investig 2012;32(12):805–15. http://dx.doi.org/10.1007/s40261-012-0008-2.
133. Bentley A, Gillard S, Spino M, et al. Cost-utility analysis of deferiprone for the treatment of β-thalassaemia patients with chronic iron overload: a UK perspective. Pharmacoeconomics 2013. http://dx.doi.org/10.1007/s40273-013-0101-2.
134. Modell B, Darlison M. Global epidemiology of haemoglobin disorders and derived service indicators. Bull World Health Organ 2008;86(6):480–7. Available at: http://www.pubmedcentral.nih.gov/articlerender.fcgi?artid52647473&tool5 pmcentrez&rendertype5abstract. Accessed December 7, 2013.

Diagnosis and Management of Iron Deficiency Anemia

Jacquelyn M. Powers, MD, George R. Buchanan, MD*

KEYWORDS

- Iron • Deficiency • Anemia • IDA • Microcytic • Therapy

KEY POINTS

- Iron deficiency anemia (IDA) affects approximately 3% of young children in the United States, whereas iron deficiency without anemia occurs in 8% to 10% of infants and children. Globally, approximately half of the world's children may have IDA, and millions of adults are affected as well.
- IDA in young children is primarily nutritional, resulting from poor iron intake due to prolonged breast-feeding and/or excessive cow milk intake, whereas in female adolescents and adults, it is usually secondary to heavy menstrual bleeding (or menorrhagia) and pregnancy. In men and postmenopausal women, its cause is primarily occult gastrointestinal blood loss.
- Manifestations of IDA in adolescents and adults include pallor, fatigue, diminished work performance, exercise intolerance, and dizziness. In children of all ages, anemia is often identified incidentally by screening or by accident when blood counts are performed for another reason.
- Initial therapy for IDA is an oral iron medication for a minimum of 3 months, while attempting to identify and correct the underlying cause. Nevertheless, firm data regarding optimal dose, duration of therapy, and monitoring of the hematologic response are unavailable.
- The administration of intravenous iron to patients who fail oral iron treatment warrants further investigation and strong consideration as a potentially safe and effective option to oral iron dosing.

HISTORY OF IRON THERAPY

In ancient Greece, iron was thought to be imparted from the mythological figure Mars and therefore associated with "force" and "strength."[1,2] It was thus primarily used therapeutically in war wounds. In the seventeenth century, Syndenham used a medicinal syrup of iron filings steeped in cold wine to reduce symptoms of chlorosis or

Disclosure Statement: The authors have nothing to disclose.
Pediatric Hematology-Oncology, University of Texas Southwestern Medical Center, 5323 Harry Hines Boulevard, Dallas, TX 75390-9063, USA
* Corresponding author.
E-mail address: george.buchanan@utsouthwestern.edu

Hematol Oncol Clin N Am 28 (2014) 729–745
http://dx.doi.org/10.1016/j.hoc.2014.04.007
0889-8588/14/$ – see front matter © 2014 Elsevier Inc. All rights reserved.

"green sickness" in young women. The treatment improved their headache, greenish nonicteric skin color, and consumption of stones and dirt. He keenly observed in 1661 that "when one gives mars in the pale color the pulse becomes at once fuller and slower, the pallor disappears and once again the face is rosy and ruddy," clearly documenting the success of a therapeutic trial of iron.[1] In the nineteenth century IDA was confirmed as the cause of chlorosis based on identification of reduced iron concentration in the blood. Use of the microscope allowed for a formal description of the corresponding hypochromic, microcytic erythrocytes on peripheral smear. In 1831, Blaud described iron treatment of chlorosis and developed the first modern-day pill—a combination of ferrous sulfate and potassium carbonate—along with specific recommendations on daily dose and duration of therapy.[1] To date, the concept of a therapeutic trial of iron, and specifically, the use of ferrous sulfate remains widely accepted by the medical community.[3]

PROBLEM OF IDA
Incidence/Prevalence

Iron deficiency is the world's most common nutrient deficiency. It affects a substantial population of women and children in both lower and higher income nations.[4] For centuries, confounders such as malnutrition and infection often masked the underlying anemia due to iron deficiency.[5] Improved nutrition and infection control later fostered better recognition of the condition, although additional confounders, such as malaria, inflammation, sickle cell disease, thalassemia, and other nutritional deficiencies, persist. Despite prevention efforts, iron deficiency and IDA are estimated to affect between 2 to 3 billion persons globally.[6,7] The highest risk groups are young women, especially those who are pregnant or postpartum, and young children.

In the United States, the widespread switch from breast-feeding to cow milk–based formulas in the 1940s resulted in a high prevalence (up to 15%) of "cow milk anemia" due to iron deficiency in young children. In 1969, the American Academy of Pediatrics (AAP) recommended the use of iron-fortified formula, which was subsequently adopted by the Women, Infants, and Children Program in the 1970s. Along with increased breast-feeding rates, the result was a decline in iron deficiency in some high-risk populations.[8] Nevertheless, IDA still occurs in approximately 3% to 7% of young children and iron deficiency without anemia has an estimated prevalence of 8% to 10%, with peak incidence from age 12 to 48 months.[8,9] Adolescent women are at risk for IDA because of heavy menstrual bleeding after onset of menarche, with an incidence of approximately 9%, and another 15% to 20% have iron deficiency without anemia.[10–12] IDA also affects 2% to 5% of pregnant women because of the expansion of red blood cell mass, which can persist postpartum due to blood loss associated with delivery.[11] The prevalence is quite low in men and postmenopausal women but increases again in the elderly.[4]

Lower income nations experience a higher prevalence of IDA due to a lack of access to meat, vegetarian diets, chronic gastrointestinal blood loss from parasitic infections, and scarcity of oral iron supplements.[4]

In this review, the optimal treatment approaches for IDA in developed countries that result from iron poor diet or blood loss are focused on, with an emphasis on young children and adolescents. However, general principles of diagnosis and therapy are applicable to patients of all ages with IDA.

CLINICAL FEATURES AND SEQUELAE OF IDA

Iron deficiency is a multisystem condition with a wide range of clinical features and sequelae, including effects on neurologic, cardiac, and immunologic functioning

(**Box 1**).[13–15] Anemia, the extreme manifestation of iron deficiency, becomes apparent after tissue iron stores are depleted. In addition to pallor, fatigue, headache, and dizziness, patients with iron deficiency often develop pica, an irresistible craving for nonfood items (ice, dirt, clay, paper, or cornstarch), which typically resolves within days to weeks after starting iron therapy.[16,17]

A driving force behind efforts to identify and prevent iron deficiency in young children is its association with lower scores on tests of mental and motor development during infancy and later at school entry, even after controlling for lower socioeconomic status.[18] Long-term studies have demonstrated poorer developmental outcome for children with IDA more than 10 years after treatment during infancy as well as identifying deficits in executive function and recognition memory almost 2 decades later.[19,20]

Iron deficiency is associated with elevated fatigue scores in young women with menorrhagia.[21] Adolescent girls with iron deficiency without anemia have improved verbal learning and memory after taking ferrous sulfate for 8 weeks compared with those receiving placebo.[22] Studies in developing countries have demonstrated increased productivity in workers with IDA who receive iron therapy versus placebo.[23] Thus, extensive evidence supports the concept that iron deficiency has a diversity of undesirable consequences.

PREVENTION AND EARLY DIAGNOSIS ARE THE IDEAL

Although IDA in children and adolescents is usually preventable, prevention strategies are often unsuccessful, as evidenced by only modest decreases in the prevalence of

---

Box 1
Manifestations and multisystem sequelae of iron deficiency

Nutritional

  Pica, pagophagia

Neurocognitive

  Reduced mental and motor function

  Poorer outcomes in executive function and recognition memory

  Visual and auditory systems' functioning

Neurologic

  Restless leg syndrome

  Neuronal hypomyelination

  Decreased neurotransmitter production

Cardiac

  Impaired myocyte function

Immunologic

  Impaired resistance to bacterial infection

Gastrointestinal

  Epithelial tissue injury (glossitis; angular stomatitis)

  Esophageal web or stricture, gastric atrophy

  Microvillus damage; protein-losing enteropathy

Hematologic

  Anemia (fatigue; diminished exercise tolerance and productivity)

iron deficiency in the United States during recent decades.[8] Once it occurs, however, prompt identification and institution of effective therapy are critical to minimize its sequelae.

Recommendations for IDA screening are summarized in **Table 1**. Screening of infants at 1 year of age is suggested but only identifies patients who are already anemic. Infants who are primarily formula fed are at low risk of IDA at 1 year of age. The transition to cow milk places them at risk for IDA during their second year of life, yet no formal screening recommendations exist in this age group.[24,25] Screening for IDA in adolescent women, another high-risk population, is not recommended by the AAP, so identification of these patients relies on the astute clinician to recognize risk factors for iron deficiency and to diagnose and treat those girls with heavy menstrual bleeding and IDA.

MANAGEMENT OF IDA

Regardless of patient age or underlying cause, 5 principles guide IDA management (**Box 2**).

Confirmation of the Diagnosis

Although a complete blood count (CBC) or a measurement of the hemoglobin concentration alone is the primary screening test used for IDA, iron deficiency progresses through several phases, with frank anemia manifested only after erythropoeisis has become markedly impaired (**Table 2**).

No specific test confirms the diagnosis of IDA in all patients, because serum ferritin may be falsely normalized/elevated and transferrin saturation may be reduced in inflammatory states.[26] The reticulocyte hemoglobin content (CHr or Ret-He) is reduced in both IDA and thalassemia trait. All of the clinical information and laboratory data must be taken into account to establish the correct diagnosis. Review of the combination of CBC, reticulocyte count, CHr or Ret-He, and peripheral smear along with serum iron, serum ferritin, and total iron binding capacity often provides evidence to support the diagnosis of IDA. However, the most convincing evidence of IDA is an increase in the hemoglobin concentration after a therapeutic trial of medicinal iron.[3]

Table 1 Screening recommendations for IDA		
Source of Recommendation	Children	Women
American Academy of Pediatrics (AAP)[24]	Universal screening at 9–12 mo; selective screening at any age for patients with risk factors	
American Academy of Family Physicians (AAFP)[68]	Follow USPSTF Guidelines	Follow USPSTF Guidelines
American College of Obstetrics & Gynecology (ACOG)[69]		All pregnant women
US Preventive Services Task Force (USPSTF) Guidelines[9]	Evidence insufficient to recommend for or against routine screening	All pregnant women
Centers for Disease Control (CDC)[10]	High-risk infants and high-risk preschool children	All nonpregnant women of childbearing age every 5–10 y

> **Box 2**
> **Principles of IDA management**
>
> 1. Confirm the diagnosis
> 2. Identify its cause
> 3. Correct or manage the primary cause
> 4. Provide iron therapy, either orally or parenterally
> 5. Confirm the success of such therapy

Other Causes of Microcytic Anemia

In patients with limited response to iron therapy and/or some normal iron measurements, other causes should be considered, such as thalassemia trait, other hemoglobinopathy, or anemia of inflammation. Iron refractory iron deficiency anemia (IRIDA), a rare form of inherited IDA described in the article by Heeney and Finberg elsewhere in this issue, should be considered in patients with lifelong IDA that is minimally responsive to oral supplementation despite good adherence to treatment and transiently responsive to parenteral iron.[27]

Identification and Management of the Primary Cause: Children and Adolescents

Iron deficiency can result from insufficient nutritional iron intake, increased requirements, malabsorption, or external bleeding. In young children, the cause is primarily nutritional. Risk factors include prematurity (as most iron transfer from mother occurs during the third trimester), exclusive breast-feeding for greater than 6 months without supplemental iron (as breast milk contains little iron), prolonged bottle-feeding, obesity, low socioeconomic status, and early, excessive, and/or prolonged intake of cow milk.[28–31] Iron in cow milk has lower bioavailability (5%–10% absorption) than human breast milk (50% absorption) and potentially interferes with duodenal absorption of iron in other foods. When consumed in excessive quantities, cow milk proteins can also damage the intestinal mucosa, leading to microvascular gastrointestinal blood loss and occasionally protein-losing enteropathy.[32,33]

In adolescent women, IDA primarily results from excessive acute and/or chronic menstrual bleeding. Given that 0.4 to 0.5 mg of iron is lost along with every 1 mL of blood, menorrhagia results in IDA that often persists or recurs. In patients with IDA not clearly caused by poor intake or heavy menstrual bleeding, other causes must

Table 2
Conventional test results in the progression of iron deficiency

	Iron Depletion	Iron-Restricted Erythropoiesis	Iron Deficiency Anemia
Hemoglobin concentration	Normal	Normal	Reduced
Mean corpuscular volume	Normal	Normal-Reduced	Reduced
Reticulocyte hemoglobin content[a]	Normal	Reduced	Reduced
Serum iron concentration	Normal	Reduced	Reduced
Serum ferritin concentration	Reduced	Reduced	Reduced
Total iron binding capacity	Normal	Increased	Increased
Soluble transferrin receptor	Normal	Increased	Increased

[a] Ret-He or CHr, the first peripheral blood count marker that becomes abnormal in iron deficiency.[70,71]

be evaluated and addressed appropriately. Specifically, gastrointestinal blood loss and/or malabsorption should be considered as well as chronic intrapulmonary bleeding or intravascular hemolysis resulting in urinary iron loss.

Identification and Management of Primary Cause: Adults

Total body iron in men is 4 g versus 3 g in women.[6] Because most women begin pregnancy with low iron reserves, the combined average iron loss during pregnancy of approximately 900 mg that results from the diversion of iron to the fetus, blood loss at delivery, and lactation often results in IDA.[11] In men and postmenopausal women, IDA is most often secondary to gastrointestinal blood loss, so it is imperative to identify and correct its source as well as provide adequate medicinal iron therapy. In adults, there is a higher incidence than in children of iron-restricted erythropoiesis during use of erythropoiesis-stimulating agents (ESAs), in which the iron supply cannot meet the increased requirements.[34] Moreover, adults have a higher incidence of "anemia of chronic disease" resulting from an elevation in the regulatory peptide hepcidin that inhibits duodenal iron absorption and renders iron stores inaccessible, as seen in chronic inflammatory conditions.[34]

Providing Iron Therapy

Regarding the first 3 management principles (see **Box 2**), there is little debate. However, recommendations in the literature about the specifics of iron therapy vary widely with regard to preparation, dosing, frequency and timing, duration, and monitoring. Recent suggestions regarding iron deficiency in young children from the AAP emphasize prevention and early diagnosis but give virtually no attention to its treatment.[24] So-called iron supplements are often prescribed at a dose that is too low and therefore ineffective, or too high, with the risk of adverse effects and poor adherence. In all patients, misguided therapy and/or poor patient education regarding IDA can result in a subpar adherence and response to therapy.

Reasons for Near Absence of Data to Inform Treatment

Many clinicians dismiss mild IDA as a benign condition with inconsequential effects, creating a false perception that research aimed to improve IDA treatment is of low priority, which has in turn resulted in a paucity of published data informing its management.[35] The scarcity of IDA clinical trials supported by governmental funding agencies, including the National Heart, Lung, and Blood Institute and National Institute of Diabetes and Digestive and Kidney Disease, is noteworthy. Moreover, limited funding from industry impedes the development of well-structured and rigorous trials aimed at answering important therapeutic questions. For example, at present, only one randomized clinical trial in the United States is comparing different oral iron medications in the treatment of IDA.[36]

ORAL IRON THERAPY
Iron Preparation

There are myriad preparations and formulations of iron, many of them available over-the-counter, causing much confusion for patients and physicians alike.[6] These agents, labeled "supplements," undergo a separate approval process by the Food and Drug Administration (FDA) and are often marketed based on slight differences involving other added vitamins and minerals (eg, B12, folate), with or without extended release properties. A 1958 review by Nathan Smith indicated that among 170 iron preparations then used in the prevention and treatment of IDA, ferrous sulfate was the least expensive and thought at the time to be the most effective.[2] To date, ferrous sulfate remains the most frequently used treatment of IDA, a testimonial to the lack of progress in the management of this condition.

Ferrous gluconate and ferrous fumarate, 2 other iron salts, have demonstrated efficacy as iron supplements for prevention and treatment of IDA.[37–40] Carbonyl iron (eg, Feosol) has also been demonstrated as a safe, effective, and inexpensive iron therapy, but it is now less frequently used.[41–43] Iron polysaccharide combinations (eg, Nulron, Niferex, NovaFerrum) are formulated as well hydrated microspheres remaining in solution over a wide range of pH values, theoretically allowing for improved absorption and tolerability.[44]

Dosing

After a specific agent is chosen, the total daily dose and divided dose schedule are based more on clinical experience than scientific evidence, but 2 basic tenets are essential: administering an adequate daily dose for a sufficient duration.[2] In persons with normal iron status, approximately 10% of dietary iron is absorbed by the duodenum, with a total daily absorptive capacity of approximately 25 mg of elemental iron.[44] Few data seem to support this estimate, and it is unclear whether it refers to the absorptive capacity following a single meal or a total daily value. However, it serves as the basis for the frequent recommendations of divided daily doses of iron therapy and refutes the concept that high single-daily doses of iron result in improved absorption and faster resolution of anemia.[45] Not surprisingly, recommended dosing in children ranges widely from 2 to 6 mg/kg/d, administered either once, twice, or 3 times daily (**Table 3**). Adult dosing suggestions vary as well from 60 to 300 mg/d of elemental iron in 2 to 4 divided doses.

In 1998, the Centers for Disease Control (CDC) suggested 3 mg/kg/d of elemental iron for treatment of IDA in children to simplify the dosing regimen and improve adherence, but the recommendation was then based on expert opinion rather than evidence from clinical trials.[46] A randomized controlled trial in rural Ghana comparing ferrous sulfate (40 mg elemental iron or approximately 3 mg/kg/d) as a single dose or as 3 divided daily doses showed similar success.[47] A study in India comparing a single daily dose of 3 mg/kg elemental iron as ferrous ascorbate to colloidal iron demonstrated correction of anemia using both agents over a 12-week study period, also supporting the efficacy of a once daily dose of iron at the lower end of the recommended range.[48]

Table 3
Recommendations for oral iron dosing in select medical textbooks

Reference	Total Daily Dose (Elemental Iron)		Number of Daily Doses
	Children	Adults	
Nelson Textbook of Pediatrics[72]	3–6 mg/kg/d		3
Rudolph's Pediatrics[73]	3–6 mg/kg/d		"Divided"
The Harriet Lane Handbook[74]	3–6 mg/kg/d	60–100 mg/dose	1 to 4
Harrison's Principles of Internal Medicine[75]		200–300 mg/d	
Nathan & Oski's Hematology of Infancy and Childhood[44]	3 mg/kg/d		1 or 3
Manual of Pediatric Hematology & Oncology[76]	4.5–6 mg/kg/d	100–200 mg daily (adolescents)	3
Hoffman: Hematology Basic Principles & Practice[17]	3 mg/kg/d	60–200 mg/d	3 or 4
Williams Hematology[11]	6 mg/kg/d	150–200 mg/d	"Divided" 3 or 4

After the daily dose is chosen, the optimal frequency and timing of dosing must be determined. Ideally, iron is recommended to be taken on an empty stomach at least 1 to 2 hours before or after meals to minimize blockade of duodenal absorption (eg, by phytates, tannins) and allow for maximum absorption. When treating young children, parents must be specifically instructed not to offer milk with the iron medication, as this will interfere with absorption. Administering iron with vitamin C may improve absorption but is probably not critical to successful therapy.[44] Acidity of the duodenal fluid facilitates iron absorption so the use of antacids or gastric surgery can impair iron absorption. Iron might have fewer adverse gastrointestinal effects if given in low dosages on an empty stomach at bedtime, although this approach has not been validated by formal studies.[45] Emphasis on the requirement of strict adherence is critical to correcting the anemia.

Patients presenting with severe IDA causing or risking heart failure should receive red cell transfusion.[49] Medicinal iron therapy as described above must follow because iron packaged in the transfused red cells is not immediately available for erythropoiesis and will not correct the depletion of body iron stores.

Hematologic Response and Duration of Therapy

Few studies have reported data regarding the specific hematologic response or adverse effect profile of oral iron therapy. One of them, a double-blind, randomized clinical trial comparing the side effects of ferrous sulfate to placebo described no differences in gastrointestinal or other adverse effects, but the hematologic response to therapy was not described.[50] A Brazilian trial of 5 mg/kg elemental iron once daily comparing carbonyl iron to ferrous sulfate demonstrated significantly higher serum ferritin levels in children receiving the former, but no significant differences in hemoglobin values were noted between the 2 groups.[43] An important study of 90 elderly patients with IDA compared responses to 3 different daily dosing regimens of elemental iron (15 mg; 50 mg; 150 mg).[51] After 2 months of therapy, hemoglobin and serum ferritin increments were similar in all 3 groups, but adverse effects and dropout rates were least in the low-dose group. This finding suggests that very low-dose iron on an empty stomach may prove effective, while having fewer adverse effects and improving adherence.

Duration of therapy is guided by the severity of anemia and the patient's response to treatment (ie, resolution of anemia and repletion of iron stores). The anemia resolves first followed by normalization of other laboratory markers of iron deficiency (**Table 4**), with measures of iron stores last to become normal.

Table 4		
Expected laboratory responses to successful iron therapy		
Test	**Time to First Response**	**Time to Sustained Normalization**
Ret He or CHr	2–3 d	2 mo
Reticulocyte count	2–3 d	6 wk
RDW	3 d	3 mo
MCV	1 wk	2 mo
Hemoglobin	1 wk	2 mo
Serum iron	1–2 h	1–2 h
Total iron binding capacity	2–3 wk	2–3 mo
Serum ferritin	1–2 wk	3 mo

Abbreviations: RDW, red cell distribution width; MCV, mean corpuscular volume.

After 3 months of therapy, it would be prudent to measure serum ferritin to confirm complete resolution of the iron deficiency (realizing that falsely normal or increased ferritin values may be the result of coexisting inflammation). In patients with suspected ongoing blood loss, malabsorption, or other circumstances where the primary cause is not controlled, follow-up is required to monitor for and treat recurrence of IDA.

Advantages and Disadvantages of Oral Iron

The major advantage of oral iron is that it is inexpensive. A major pitfall, however, is poor adherence, which inevitably results in treatment failure in an appreciable percentage of patients irrespective of the cause of IDA. Families of young children may report refusal and spitting up doses due to the poor taste of many iron preparations. Patients of any age may complain of adverse effects, which are primarily gastrointestinal (constipation, dark stools, nausea, vomiting, abdominal pain). The adverse effects of iron preparations, need for prolonged daily therapy, inconvenience, and perceived "benign" nature of the condition are singly or in combination often responsible for treatment failure. A final word of caution applies to the risk of accidental ingestion and overdose when young children are in the household, as iron medications are among the most frequent cause of this complication.[9]

INTRAVENOUS IRON THERAPY

In the 1950s, high-molecular-weight iron dextran (HMWID) was the first intravenous iron formulation used in the United States. Multiple adverse effects, including reports of anaphylactic reactions, led to restricted use. However, since the early 1990s, several new intravenous preparations have been developed, tested, and FDA approved.[52–55]

Indications for Intravenous Iron

Intravenous iron should be used as first-line therapy for most patients with iron-restricted erythropoiesis caused by elevated levels of hepcidin as well as patients receiving chronic dialysis and ESAs.[34,56] Given the adverse effects or poor efficacy of oral iron in patients with gastrointestinal disorders, such as celiac disease or inflammatory bowel disease, intravenous iron may be appropriate first-line therapy.[57,58] It should also be considered in patients with IDA not responding to oral iron, whether due to poor compliance, intolerance of adverse effects, malabsorption, or ongoing blood loss.

Intravenous Iron Preparations

Intravenous iron formulations differ in administration, dosing, adverse effects, cost, and FDA indication, all which must be taken into account when considering which preparation is most appropriate (**Table 5**). The patient's likely requirement for ongoing iron therapy is also a consideration.

One of "newer" intravenous preparations is low-molecular-weight iron dextran (LMWID; INFeD), which has a markedly improved safety profile compared with the HMWID that was used several decades ago.[53] Until recently, LMWID was the only formulation that allowed for a total drug infusion (TDI) at a single visit, with up to 1000 mg administered over 1 to 4 hours. More rapid administration increases the risk of acute infusion reactions due to the transient effects of labile or free iron release.[59] Despite the lower risk of reactions with LMWID in contrast to HMWID, a test dose is still required before full-dose infusion.[60]

Table 5
Intravenous iron preparations available in the United States

Generic (Trade) Name	Ferric Gluconate (Ferrlecit)	Iron Sucrose (Venofer)	Low-Molecular-Weight Iron Dextran (INFeD)	Ferumoxytol (Feraheme)	Ferric Carboxymaltose (Injectafer)	Iron Isomaltoside 1000 (Monofer)
Manufacturer	Sanofi Aventis Inc	American Regent Inc	Watson Pharmaceuticals Inc	AMAG Pharmaceuticals	American Regent Inc	Pharamcosmos A/S
FDA indication (adult)	Patients with chronic kidney disease on dialysis + ESAs	Patients with chronic kidney disease	Patients in whom oral iron administration is unsatisfactory or impossible	Patients with chronic kidney disease	Patients with intolerance or unsatisfactory response to oral iron; non-dialysis-dependent chronic kidney disease	Patients in whom oral iron preparations are ineffective or cannot be used; clinical need for rapid iron delivery
FDA approved (pediatrics)	Yes, >6 y	Yes, >2 y	Yes, >4 mo	No	No	No
Maximum approved dose	125 mg	200 mg	100 mg	510 mg	750 mg	20 mg/kg
TDI possible	No	No	Yes (Europe)	Yes	Yes (Europe)	Yes
TDI infusion time	60 min	2–5 min	60 min	15–60 min	15 min	30 min (≤1000 mg) 60 min (>1000 mg)
Test dose required	No	No	Yes	No	No	No
Adverse effects	Hypotension; ab pain, N/V	Hypotension; ab pain, N/V	Allergic; anaphylactic	Anaphylaxis; hypotension	Anaphylaxis; N/V, hypertension, flushing	Anaphylaxis; ab pain, N/V
Black box warning	No	No	Yes	No	No	No
Iron concentration	12.5 mg/mL	20 mg/mL	50 mg/mL	30 mg/mL	30 mg/mL	100 mg/mL
Vial size	5 mL	5 mL	2 mL	17 mL	2 mL	1, 5 and 10 mL

Adapted from Auerbach M, Ballard H. Clinical use of intravenous iron: administration, efficacy, and safety. Hematology Am Soc Hematol Educ Program 2010;2010:340.

Two intravenous iron polysaccharide preparations, ferric gluconate (Ferrlecit) and iron sucrose (Venofer), lack the dextran moiety of LMWID and therefore may have a lower incidence of infusion reactions.[60,61] Both formulations are administered over a relatively short period of time. However, doses exceeding more than 250 to 300 mg result in high rates of infusion reactions due to free iron release from the less tightly bound carbohydrate carriers and are characterized by hypotension, chest and abdominal pain, vomiting, and diarrhea.[59,62] Hence, iron polysaccharide formulations may require multiple outpatient infusion visits for patients who need a larger total repletion dose.

Ferumoxytol (Feraheme) was approved in 2009 for the treatment of IDA in patients with chronic kidney disease. It is a colloidal iron oxide, coated with a semisynthetic carbohydrate shell that minimizes immunologic reactivity (ie, lower free iron release) compared with other agents, thus eliminating the need for a test dose.[63] The drug is phagocytosed by macrophages and then slowly released into circulation after administration.[60] An advantage over other intravenous preparations is the ability to administer a TDI over 15 minutes.[59]

Two formulations recently licensed for use in the United States are ferric carboxymaltose (Injectafer) and iron isomaltoside 1000 (Monofer). They are approved for rapid administration of a TDI at a single visit without the need for a test dose. Although ferric carboxymaltose is dosed at 15 mg/kg (maximum 750 mg), iron isomaltoside 1000 is dosed at 20 mg/kg with no maximum.[56] Unlike ferumoxytol, ferric carboxymaltose has been FDA approved for adults who have intolerance or unsatisfactory response to oral iron and has demonstrated safety and efficacy superior to oral iron.[62]

Dosing and Administration

Dosing of intravenous iron is based on the patient's initial hemoglobin value, targeted "ideal" hemoglobin concentration, and weight (with a maximum dose as based on each manufacturer's guidelines). Administration of a test dose is required for some intravenous formulations as described above. The most commonly reported adverse reactions for intravenous iron preparations include urticaria, dyspnea, pruritis, tachycardia, chest discomfort, chills, and arthralgia. Premedication with diphenhydramine, acetaminophen, and/or steroids is not required, but should be considered in patients with a history of other drug allergies or asthma.[64]

Intravenous Iron in Children

Although most studies of intravenous iron include only adults, recent research has confirmed that intravenous iron may also be safely administered to children with IDA.[57] For example, repeated doses of intravenous iron sucrose in 38 children with IDA unresponsive to oral iron were successful with no or minimal toxicity.[55] A more recent study of 31 children from the same center reported that a TDI of intravenous LMWID was both well tolerated and effective, although some patients with ongoing blood loss required additional infusions.[64] A case series of 6 children with gastrointestinal disorders demonstrated the safe administration of ferumoxytol as well.[60]

Oral Versus Intravenous Iron

A substantial advantage of intravenous iron therapy is that it bypasses the need for oral intake and intestinal absorption of medicinal iron (**Table 6**). Some parenteral preparations also offer the option of a single TDI, which eliminates the need for frequent repeated infusions or a prolonged course of oral iron medication with its many disadvantages, thereby preventing treatment failure due to poor adherence. It seems to be an excellent choice for patients whose IDA is refractory despite best efforts at

Table 6
Comparison of oral versus intravenous iron administration

	Oral Iron	Intravenous Iron
Indications	Supplementation for patients at risk for IDA Nutritional IDA IDA due to menorrhagia IDA due to pregnancy	Functional iron deficiency (on ESAs) Poor iron mobilization (inflammation; IRIDA) Gastrointestinal conditions (irritable bowel disease, celiac disease) Oral iron treatment failure/intolerance
Adverse effects	Primarily gastrointestinal (dose-dependent)	Primarily related to infusion reaction
Duration of therapy	Minimum 3 mo, often longer due to poor compliance	If primary cause addressed, only single infusion/visit necessary
Cost	Inexpensive but additional follow-up visits necessary	Expensive, primarily due to drug infusion costs
Quality of life	Dependent on adverse effects, resolution of anemia, multiple visits, laboratory testing	Potential one time infusion with no long-term compliance issues

successful treatment with oral iron preparations. Ideally, in patients for whom the underlying cause can be corrected, a one-time TDI of intravenous iron could essentially "cure" the IDA, relieving patients and families of the need for ongoing visits and repeated laboratory monitoring.

The principal disadvantages of intravenous iron agents include the substantial costs of the drug and the infusion. Although serious adverse effects are now infrequent, they may still occur and require close monitoring for all patients.

FUTURE RESEARCH
Need for Pragmatic Therapeutic Trials

Pragmatic, low-cost, randomized controlled trials focused on the treatment of IDA, with regard to iron preparation, dose, adverse effects, adherence, and total length of therapy, are badly needed. Such patient-centered trials would test the effectiveness of an intervention in the broad spectrum of everyday clinical settings to maximize generalizability of the results.[65] The comparative effectiveness of interventions used in routine practice would allow for implementation of cost analyses, which could in turn inform policymakers and health care providers about a treatment's cost in real-life situations and provide clinicians a tried and true approach to the successful treatment of their IDA patients.[66]

Few, if any, studies have directly compared oral versus intravenous iron for the treatment of patients with IDA, regardless of age or cause. Given the numerous limitations of oral iron therapy, the utilization of intravenous iron treatment regimens must be further explored.[61] A well-designed study of up-front intravenous versus oral iron therapy in young children and adolescents, which evaluates treatment response, cost analysis, and quality of life measures, could be of groundbreaking importance.[67]

SUMMARY

- Iron deficiency results in multiorgan sequelae, thus warranting its prevention. Anemia due to iron deficiency requires prompt and appropriate treatment.

- The principles of iron therapy include (1) confirmation of IDA, (2) identification of its cause, (3) correcting or managing its etiology, (4) providing appropriate iron therapy, either orally or parenterally, and (5) confirming resolution of iron deficiency and IDA. Adequate iron therapy requires an adequate dose for a sufficient time period.
- In the future, clinical trials regarding dose, monitoring strategy, and total duration of iron therapy are necessary in diverse patient populations.
- New intravenous iron preparations with improved safety profiles offer attractive options for optimal management of IDA in both the pediatric and the adult populations, including the benefit of a single TDI.

REFERENCES

1. Christian HA. A sketch of the history of the treatment of chlorosis with iron. Med Library Hist J 1903;1(3):176–80.
2. Smith NJ. Iron as a therapeutic agent in pediatric practice. J Pediatr 1958;53(1): 37–50.
3. Oski FA. Iron deficiency in infancy and childhood. N Engl J Med 1993;329(3): 190–3.
4. de Benoist B, Hempstead R. Iron deficiency anaemia: assessment, prevention, and control. A guide for programme managers. Geneva, Switzerland: World Health Organization; 2001.
5. Pearson HA. History of pediatric hematology oncology. Pediatr Res 2002;52(6): 979–92.
6. Rockey DC. Treatment of iron deficiency. Gastroenterology 2006;130(4):1367–8.
7. McLean E, Cogswell M, Egli I, et al. Worldwide prevalence of anaemia, WHO vitamin and mineral nutrition information system, 1993-2005. Public Health Nutr 2009;12(4):444–54.
8. Brotanek JM, Gosz J, Weitzman M, et al. Secular trends in the prevalence of iron deficiency among US toddlers, 1976-2002. Arch Pediatr Adolesc Med 2008; 162(4):374–81.
9. Screening for iron deficiency anemia–including iron supplementation for children and pregnant women: U.S. Preventive Services Task Force. 2006.
10. Centers for Disease Control and Prevention (CDC). Iron deficiency–United States, 1999-2000. MMWR Morb Mortal Wkly Rep 2002;51(40):897–9.
11. Beutler E. Disorders of iron metabolism. In: Lichtman MA, Kipps TJ, Seligsohn U, et al, editors. Williams hematology. 8th edition. New York: The McGraw-Hill Companies; 2010. Available at: http://accessmedicine.mhmedical.com/content. aspx?bookid=358&Sectionid=39835860. Accessed November 4, 2013.
12. Bar-Or D. Screening for iron deficiency. N Engl J Med 1982;307(22):1405–6.
13. Algarin C, Peirano P, Garrido M, et al. Iron deficiency anemia in infancy: long-lasting effects on auditory and visual system functioning. Pediatr Res 2003; 53(2):217–23.
14. Lozoff B, Beard J, Connor J, et al. Long-lasting neural and behavioral effects of iron deficiency in infancy. Nutr Rev 2006;64(5 Pt 2):S34–43 [discussion: S72–91].
15. Kabakus N, Ayar A, Yoldas TK, et al. Reversal of iron deficiency anemia-induced peripheral neuropathy by iron treatment in children with iron deficiency anemia. J Trop Pediatr 2002;48(4):204–9.
16. Starn AL, Udall JN Jr. Iron deficiency anemia, pica, and restless legs syndrome in a teenage girl. Clin Pediatr (Phila) 2008;47(1):83–5.

17. Brittenham GM. Disorders of iron homeostasis: iron deficiency and overload. In: Hoffman R, Benz EJ, Silberstein LE, et al, editors. Hematology: basic principles and practice. 6th edition. Philadelphia: Elsevier; 2012. p. 441–2.

18. Lozoff B, Jimenez E, Wolf AW. Long-term developmental outcome of infants with iron deficiency. N Engl J Med 1991;325(10):687–94.

19. Lozoff B, Jimenez E, Hagen J, et al. Poorer behavioral and developmental outcome more than 10 years after treatment for iron deficiency in infancy. Pediatrics 2000;105(4):E51.

20. Lukowski AF, Koss M, Burden MJ, et al. Iron deficiency in infancy and neurocognitive functioning at 19 years: evidence of long-term deficits in executive function and recognition memory. Nutr Neurosci 2010;13(2):54–70.

21. Wang W, Bourgeois T, Klima J, et al. Iron deficiency and fatigue in adolescent females with heavy menstrual bleeding. Haemophilia 2013;19(2):225–30.

22. Bruner AB, Joffe A, Duggan AK, et al. Randomised study of cognitive effects of iron supplementation in non-anaemic iron-deficient adolescent girls. Lancet 1996;348(9033):992–6.

23. Edgerton VR, Gardner GW, Ohira Y, et al. Iron-deficiency anaemia and its effect on worker productivity and activity patterns. Br Med J 1979;2(6204): 1546–9.

24. Baker RD, Greer FR. Diagnosis and prevention of iron deficiency and iron-deficiency anemia in infants and young children (0-3 years of age). Pediatrics 2010;126(5):1040–50.

25. Buchanan GR. The tragedy of iron deficiency during infancy and early childhood. J Pediatr 1999;135(4):413–5.

26. Brugnara C, Adamson J, Auerbach M, et al. Iron deficiency: what are the future trends in diagnostics and therapeutics? Clin Chem 2013;59(5):740–5.

27. Buchanan GR, Sheehan RG. Malabsorption and defective utilization of iron in three siblings. J Pediatr 1981;98(5):723–8.

28. Male C, Persson LA, Freeman V, et al. Prevalence of iron deficiency in 12-mo-old infants from 11 European areas and influence of dietary factors on iron status (Euro-Growth study). Acta Paediatr 2001;90(5):492–8.

29. Moy RJ. Prevalence, consequences and prevention of childhood nutritional iron deficiency: a child public health perspective. Clin Lab Haematol 2006;28(5): 291–8.

30. Brotanek JM, Gosz J, Weitzman M, et al. Iron deficiency in early childhood in the United States: risk factors and racial/ethnic disparities. Pediatrics 2007;120(3): 568–75.

31. Brotanek JM, Halterman JS, Auinger P, et al. Iron deficiency, prolonged bottle-feeding, and racial/ethnic disparities in young children. Arch Pediatr Adolesc Med 2005;159(11):1038–42.

32. Nickerson HJ, Silberman T, Park RW, et al. Treatment of iron deficiency anemia and associated protein-losing enteropathy in children. J Pediatr Hematol Oncol 2000;22(1):50–4.

33. Salstrom JL, Kent M, Liang X, et al. Toddlers with anasarca and severe anemia: a lesson in preventive medicine. Curr Opin Pediatr 2012;24(1):129–33.

34. Goodnough LT, Nemeth E, Ganz T. Detection, evaluation, and management of iron-restricted erythropoiesis. Blood 2010;116(23):4754–61.

35. Buchanan GR. Paucity of clinical trials in iron deficiency: lessons learned from study of VLBW infants. Pediatrics 2013;131(2):e582–4.

36. Clinicaltrials.gov. Comparison of NovaFerrum® vs Ferrous Sulfate treatment in young children with nutritional iron deficiency anemia (BESTIRON). 2013. Available

at: http://www.clinicaltrials.gov/ct2/show/NCT01904864?term=iron+deficiency+ anemia+children&recr=Open&rank=1. Accessed November 21, 2013.

37. Radtke H, Tegtmeier J, Rocker L, et al. Daily doses of 20 mg of elemental iron compensate for iron loss in regular blood donors: a randomized, double-blind, placebo-controlled study. Transfusion 2004;44(10):1427–32.

38. Jaber L, Rigler S, Taya A, et al. Iron polymaltose versus ferrous gluconate in the prevention of iron deficiency anemia of infancy. J Pediatr Hematol Oncol 2010; 32(8):585–8.

39. Hurrell R. Use of ferrous fumarate to fortify foods for infants and young children. Nutr Rev 2010;68(9):522–30.

40. Hirve S, Bhave S, Bavdekar A, et al. Low dose 'Sprinkles'– an innovative approach to treat iron deficiency anemia in infants and young children. Indian Pediatr 2007;44(2):91–100.

41. Gordeuk VR, Brittenham GM, McLaren CE, et al. Carbonyl iron therapy for iron deficiency anemia. Blood 1986;67(3):745–52.

42. Gordeuk VR, Brittenham GM, Hughes M, et al. High-dose carbonyl iron for iron deficiency anemia: a randomized double-blind trial. Am J Clin Nutr 1987;46(6): 1029–34.

43. Farias ILG, Colpo E, Botton SR, et al. Carbonyl iron reduces anemia and improves effectiveness of treatment in under six-year-old children. Revista Brasileira de Hematologia e Hemoterapia 2009;31(3):125–31.

44. Andrews NC, Ullrich CK, Fleming MD. Disorders of iron metabolism and sideroblastic anemia. In: Orkin SH, Nathan DG, Ginsburg D, et al, editors. Nathan and Oski's hematology of infancy and childhood. 7th edition. Philadelphia: Sunders Elsevier; 2009. p. 521–42.

45. Sandoval C, Jayabose S, Eden AN. Trends in diagnosis and management of iron deficiency during infancy and early childhood. Hematol Oncol Clin North Am 2004;18(6):1423–38.

46. Recommendations to prevent and control iron deficiency in the united states: centers for disease control and prevention. MMWR Recomm Rep 1998;47:1–29.

47. Zlotkin S, Arthur P, Antwi KY, et al. Randomized, controlled trial of single versus 3-times-daily ferrous sulfate drops for treatment of anemia. Pediatrics 2001; 108(3):613–6.

48. Yewale VN, Dewan B. Treatment of iron deficiency anemia in children: a comparative study of ferrous ascorbate and colloidal iron. Indian J Pediatr 2013;80(5):385–90.

49. Kwiatkowski JL, West TB, Heidary N, et al. Severe iron deficiency anemia in young children. J Pediatr 1999;135(4):514–6.

50. Reeves JD, Yip R. Lack of adverse side effects of oral ferrous sulfate therapy in 1-year-old infants. Pediatrics 1985;75(2):352–5.

51. Rimon E, Kagansky N, Kagansky M, et al. Are we giving too much iron? Low-dose iron therapy is effective in octogenarians. Am J Med 2005;118(10):1142–7.

52. Chertow GM, Mason PD, Vaage-Nilsen O, et al. Update on adverse drug events associated with parenteral iron. Nephrol Dial Transplant 2006;21(2):378–82.

53. Chertow GM, Mason PD, Vaage-Nilsen O, et al. On the relative safety of parenteral iron formulations. Nephrol Dial Transplant 2004;19(6):1571–5.

54. Pinsk V, Levy J, Moser A, et al. Efficacy and safety of intravenous iron sucrose therapy in a group of children with iron deficiency anemia. Isr Med Assoc J 2008;10(5):335–8.

55. Crary SE, Hall K, Buchanan GR. Intravenous iron sucrose for children with iron deficiency failing to respond to oral iron therapy. Pediatr Blood Cancer 2011; 56(4):615–9.

56. Gozzard D. When is high-dose intravenous iron repletion needed? Assessing new treatment options. Drug Des Devel Ther 2011;5:51–60.

57. Mamula P, Piccoli DA, Peck SN, et al. Total dose intravenous infusion of iron dextran for iron-deficiency anemia in children with inflammatory bowel disease. J Pediatr Gastroenterol Nutr 2002;34(3):286–90.

58. Gasche C, Berstad A, Befrits R, et al. Guidelines on the diagnosis and management of iron deficiency and anemia in inflammatory bowel diseases. Inflamm Bowel Dis 2007;13(12):1545–53.

59. Auerbach M, Strauss W, Auerbach S, et al. Safety and efficacy of total dose infusion of 1,020 mg of ferumoxytol administered over 15 min. Am J Hematol 2013; 88(11):944–7.

60. Hassan N, Cahill J, Rajasekaran S, et al. Ferumoxytol infusion in pediatric patients with gastrointestinal disorders: first case series. Ann Pharmacother 2011;45(12):e63.

61. Auerbach M. Should intravenous iron be upfront therapy for iron deficiency anemia? Pediatr Blood Cancer 2011;56(4):511–2.

62. Onken JE, Bregman DB, Harrington RA, et al. A multicenter, randomized, active-controlled study to investigate the efficacy and safety of intravenous ferric carboxymaltose in patients with iron deficiency anemia. Transfusion 2014;54: 306–15.

63. Vadhan-Raj S, Strauss W, Ford D, et al. Efficacy and safety of IV ferumoxytol for adults with iron deficiency anemia previously unresponsive to or unable to tolerate oral iron. Am J Hematol 2014;89:7–12.

64. Plummer ES, Crary SE, McCavit TL, et al. Intravenous low molecular weight iron dextran in children with iron deficiency anemia unresponsive to oral iron. Pediatr Blood Cancer 2013;60(11):1747–52.

65. Patsopoulos NA. A pragmatic view on pragmatic trials. Dialogues Clin Neurosci 2011;13(2):217–24.

66. Naim M, Hunter J. Intravenous iron replacement - management in general practice. Aust Fam Physician 2010;39(11):839–41.

67. Forman E. Goodbye oral iron therapy? Pediatr Blood Cancer 2013;60(11): 1731.

68. (AAFP) AAoFP. Iron deficiency anemia. 2006. Available at: http://www.aafp.org/patient-care/clinical-recommendations/all/iron-deficiency-anemia.html. Accessed December 15, 2013.

69. American College of Obstetricians and Gynecologists. ACOG Practice Bulletin no. 95: anemia in pregnancy. Obstet Gynecol 2008;112(1):201–7.

70. Brugnara C, Schiller B, Moran J. Reticulocyte hemoglobin equivalent (Ret He) and assessment of iron-deficient states. Clin Lab Haematol 2006;28(5): 303–8.

71. Mast AE, Blinder MA, Dietzen DJ. Reticulocyte hemoglobin content. Am J Hematol 2008;83(4):307–10.

72. Lerner NB, Sills R. Iron deficiency anemia. In: Kliegman RM, Stanton BF, Gemelll JW, et al, editors. Nelson textbook of pediatrics. 19th edition. Philadelphia: Elsevier; 2011. p. 1658.

73. Heeney MM. Anemia. In: Rudolph AM, Lister GE, First LR, et al, editors. Rudolph's pediatrics. New York: McGraw-Hill; 2011. Available at: http://accesspediatrics.mhmedical.com/content.aspx?bookid=455. Accessed November 4, 2013.

74. Lee CK, Tschudy MM, Arcara KM. Drug doses. In: Tschudy MM, Arcara KM, editors. The Harriet Lane handbook: a manual for pediatric house officers. 19th edition. Philadelphia: Elsevier; 2011. p. 830.

75. Adamson JW. Iron deficiency and other hypoproliferative anemias. In: Longo DL, Fauci AS, Kasper DL, et al, editors. Harrison's principles of internal medicine. 18th edition. The McGraw-Hill Companies, Inc; 2012. Available at: http://access medicine.mhmedical.com/content.aspx?bookid=331&Sectionid=40726841. Accessed November 4, 2013.
76. Lanzkowsky P. Iron-deficiency anemia. In: Lanzkowsky P, editor. Manual of pediatric hematology and oncology. 5th edition. Philadelphia: Elsevier; 2011. p. 38–57.

Use of Magnetic Resonance Imaging to Monitor Iron Overload

John C. Wood, MD, PhD[a,b,*]

KEYWORDS

- Iron overload • Thalassemia • Sickle cell disease • Chelation
- Magnetic resonance imaging • Iron • Liver • Heart

KEY POINTS

- Serum ferritin and transferrin saturation remain valuable in tracking the therapeutic response to iron-removal therapies.
- These inexpensive techniques have many shortcomings that preclude using them safely as sole monitors for chelator efficacy.
- Magnetic resonance imaging has become the de facto gold standard for tracking iron levels in the body because it is accurate, reproducible, and well tolerated by patients, and can track iron levels in different organs of the body.
- The latter characteristic is important because the mechanisms and kinetics of iron uptake and clearance vary across somatic organs.
- The author's clinical practice is presented as a reference, but individual experiences will still be colored by local expertise as the technologies continue to mature and be more widely distributed.

MONITORING TRANSFUSION BURDEN

Each unit of packed red blood cells (PRBCs) contains between 200 and 250 mg of iron. In fact, the iron can be calculated from the hematocrit (Hct) using the following relationship:

$$\text{Transfusional iron intake (mg/kg)} = \text{blood volume (mL/kg)} \times \text{Hct} \times 1.08 \text{ mg/mL} \quad (1)$$

---

[a] Department of Pediatrics, Children's Hospital, Los Angeles, Keck School of Medicine, University of Southern California, 4650 Sunset Boulevard, Los Angeles, CA 90027, USA; [b] Department of Radiology, Children's Hospital, Los Angeles, Keck School of Medicine, University of Southern California, 4650 Sunset Boulevard, Los Angeles, CA 90027, USA
* Cardiovascular MRI Laboratory, Children's Hospital Los Angeles, 4650 Sunset Boulevard, MS #34, Los Angeles, CA 90027.
E-mail address: jwood@chla.usc.edu

Hematol Oncol Clin N Am 28 (2014) 747–764
http://dx.doi.org/10.1016/j.hoc.2014.04.002
0889-8588/14/$ – see front matter © 2014 Elsevier Inc. All rights reserved.

where Hct is calculated from the PRBCs provided by the blood bank.[1] The volume of transfused blood in 1 year can be converted to a predicted change in liver iron concentration (LIC) if no chelation is taken, using the following equation[2]:

$$\Delta LIC = \text{Transfusion iron intake}/10.6 \qquad (2)$$

Thus a patient receiving 150 mL/kg/y of PRBCs having an Hct of 70% would increase the liver iron by 10 mg/g in the absence of iron chelation. As a rule of thumb, each 15 mL/kg transfusion will raise liver iron by approximately 1 mg/g dry weight.

Therefore, tracking transfusional iron exposure is a logical and conceptually simple way of predicting iron chelation needs, a priori. It is clearly useful in deciding when to initiate iron chelation therapy. Systematic intensification of transfusion requirements, such as may occur during hepatitis C treatment, should prompt preemptive changes in iron chelation. However, there are 2 major limitations to using transfusional burden to adjust chelation. In practice, values may be difficult to track because amounts released from the blood bank are systematically larger than are given to the patients. More importantly, there are complicated interactions between transfusion iron rate and chelator efficacy that may be patient and disease specific, creating differences between predicted and observed response to therapy.

SERUM MARKERS OF IRON OVERLOAD

Ferritin is an intracellular iron-storage protein that is essential for all living cells because it maintains labile cellular iron levels within a safe range while protecting cells against iron deficiency in the future. The circulating serum ferritin pool mostly arises from the liver and reticuloendothelial systems, and its biological role is unclear. The relationship between serum ferritin and total body iron stores is complicated. Correlation coefficients between ferritin and liver iron concentration are typically around 0.7, leaving 50% of the variability unexplained.[3,4] More importantly, the confidence intervals for predicting LIC values from serum ferritin measurements are enormous. A patient having a serum ferritin level of 1500 ng/mL could have a LIC as low as 3 or as high as 30 mg/g dry weight. As a result, toxicity thresholds based on serum ferritin levels can be dangerously misleading.

Serum ferritin may be so unreliable because it is an acute-phase reactant[5] that rises sharply with inflammation. The liver is the major source of circulating ferritin, and even minor liver insults will sharply increase serum ferritin.[6] By contrast, ascorbate deficiency leads to inappropriately low serum ferritin values relative to iron stores.[7] Lastly, serum ferritin levels depend on the transfusion rate in addition to the body's iron stores. Nontransfused iron-overloaded patients, such as those with β-thalassemia intermedia, have much lower ferritin values for a given total-body iron concentration.[8]

Intrapatient trends in serum ferritin improve its predictive value.[8] The author typically measures serum ferritin values with every transfusion, and trend median values over a period of 3 to 6 months. Nonetheless, ferritin and LIC trends remain discordant more than 30% of the time.[9] Periods of discordance can span months to years.[9]

Despite its limitations, serum ferritin is undoubtedly the world's most widely used method for tracking iron stores because of its low cost and universal availability. **Box 1** summarizes guidelines for improved use of serum ferritin to trend iron overload.

Transferrin saturation is also an important and widely available serologic marker of iron balance. It represents the earliest and most specific marker of primary hemochromatosis, and is a key screening marker in all diagnostic algorithms for this disease.[10] Increased transferrin saturation can also be used as an indicator to initiate iron

<table>
<tr><td>
Box 1
Guidelines for use of serum ferritin to monitor iron balance
</td></tr>
<tr><td>

1. Measure serum ferritin every or every other transfusion visit for transfused patients and quarterly for nontransfused patients

2. Calculate median values over 3- to 6-month intervals for trends

3. Monitor and prevent ascorbate deficiency

4. Anchor each serum ferritin trends to LIC assessments at a minimum of every 2 years

5. Repeat MRI if trends in serum ferritin are incongruent with reported patient compliance or other clinical assessments

</td></tr>
</table>

chelation therapy in thalassemia intermedia[11,12] in addition to all secondary hemochromatosis syndromes.

Many chronically transfused patients have fully saturated transferrin, making it uninformative for short-term and mid-term assessment of chelation efficiency. The prevalence of circulating non–transferrin-bound iron (NTBI) increases dramatically once transferrin saturation exceeds 85%.[13] Thus, desaturating transferrin to less than 85% is a reasonable long-term target for iron chelation therapy in transfusional siderosis syndromes. However, from a practical perspective, transferrin saturation cannot be accurately assessed in the presence of circulating chelator so patients must hold their iron chelation for 24 hours before their blood draw, limiting the practicality of frequent monitoring by this method. The author recommends annual screening of transferrin saturation in chronically transfused patients, in line with other screening laboratories.

MEASUREMENT OF LIVER IRON CONCENTRATION

The liver accounts for approximately 70% to 80% of the total-body iron stores in iron-overloaded patients. As a result, changes in liver iron accurately predict the balance between transfusional burden and iron-removal therapies.[2,14] LIC exceeding 17 mg/g dry weight is associated with iron-mediated hepatocellular damage.[15] Patients with LIC values above this threshold are also at increased risk for cardiac iron overload.[14,16–18] Long-term liver siderosis is associated in increased risk of hepatocellular carcinoma in patients with hereditary hemochromatosis.[19] Hepatocellular carcinoma is also becoming a leading cause of death in iron-loaded adults with thalassemia syndromes,[20,21] even in patients who are hepatitis C negative.[8]

Whereas increased LIC places patients at particular danger for iron-overload complications, there is no "safe" LIC threshold below which cardiac and endocrine iron accumulation does not occur.[22] The reason for this apparent paradox is that many chronically transfused patients have fully saturated transferrin, regardless of their LIC.[13] Patients who miss chelator doses expose their extrahepatic organs to unrestricted uptake of labile iron species.[23]

Despite its limitations, LIC remains the best single metric for tracking chelator response and dosing adjustments. At most major thalassemia and sickle cell disease (SCD) centers, it is measured annually to guide chelation therapy.

Liver Biopsy

Traditionally, LIC was measured by ultrasound-guided transcutaneous needle biopsy. Biopsy has the advantage of providing both histologic assessment of liver damage and iron quantification. The complication rate is acceptable, typically about 0.5%, but life-threatening hemorrhages occur.[24] The single greatest limitation is the spatial heterogeneity of tissue iron deposition in the liver that can result in high sampling variability, even in the absence of significant liver disease. When significant fibrosis is present, the coefficient of variability can exceed 40%, making biopsy essentially useless for tracking response to therapy.[25–27] Following collection from a cutting needle, liver samples are fixed in formaldehyde and sent fresh or paraffin-embedded to special laboratories for quantification. Iron quantification is generally performed using tissue digestion in nitric acid followed by either atomic absorption or inductively coupled mass spectrometry. These assays have a coefficient of variation of around 12%, independent of the sampling variability.[28] Values are reported as mg/g dry weight of tissue. Paraffin-embedded specimens must be dewaxed with organic solvents before digestion. This process lowers the tissue dry weight because it removes membrane lipids, raising the apparent iron concentration.[29] Because of its known systematic and random errors, cost, and invasiveness, liver biopsy can no longer be considered the gold standard for LIC assessment, and should not be used except when tissue histology is necessary for diagnosis.

Computed Tomography

Iron increases x-ray attenuation proportionally to its concentration. The ability of carefully calibrated quantitative computed tomography (qCT) measurements to measure liver iron has been known for decades.[30] Two basic approaches used are single-energy and dual-energy techniques.

In single-energy techniques, a low-dose qCT scan is performed at a middle hepatic level and the liver attenuation is compared with an external phantom control. The phantom need not be iron-based; it is simply necessary to correct for imperfections in the x-ray beam. The chief limitation of this approach is that changes in attenuation caused by iron are small in comparison with normal attenuation fluctuations. Thus single-energy qCT cannot accurately track LIC changes for LIC values less than 7 mg/g dry weight, and is less accurate than magnetic resonance imaging (MRI) measurements for LIC values less than 15 or 20 mg/g.[31,32] By contrast, qCT is fairly robust for severe iron overload.

In dual-energy techniques, measurements are performed at low and high x-ray beam energies, and the difference is used to predict the amount of iron. Non–iron-loaded tissue has similar attenuation values at both field strengths, and is suppressed when the difference is calculated. Although this potentially offers better discrimination at low iron concentrations, it requires higher radiation exposure to achieve it. Feasibility was demonstrated in animal studies nearly 2 decades ago,[30,32] but there have been no validation studies performed using modern equipment.

Magnetic Detectors

Tissue iron is paramagnetic. Consequently, devices that measure the magnetic properties of liver can quantify liver iron. The first devices to accomplish this used superconducting magnetic coils and were known as superconducting quantum interference devices (SQUIDs).[33,34] Although reasonably accurate, these devices are expensive, require specialized expertise for measurement acquisition and device maintenance, and can only quantitate iron in the liver and spleen. As a result, only 4 SQUID devices suitable for LIC quantification are operational worldwide. More inexpensive devices that operate at room temperature could potentially become practical in the future, but remain research tools for the present.[35]

Magnetic Resonance Imaging

MRI can also be used to quantify iron overload. It does not measure liver iron directly, but the effect of liver iron on water protons as they diffuse in the magnetically inhomogeneous environment caused by iron deposition.[36] The principles are simple. The scanner transmits energy into the body in the form of microwaves, waits a period of time, and then actively recalls this energy as microwaves that are received by an antenna or "coil." The longer the scanner waits before recalling an echo, the less energy returns. This process is known as relaxation, and is characterized by the relaxation rates R2 and R2* (measured in Hz). These rates are simply the mathematical inverse of the characteristic relaxation times, T2 and T2* (measured in milliseconds). The higher is the iron concentration, the higher the relaxation rates and the shorter the relaxation times. The difference between R2 and R2* depends on how the scanner forms the echo. R2* is the parameter measured for gradient-formed echoes but R2 is the parameter measured if radiofrequency pulses are used to form the echo (spin echo).

The first large study validating MRI as a means to quantify liver iron used a specific protocol to measure liver R2.[37] The R2 calibration curve was curvilinear and exhibited limits of agreement of −56% to 56%. Much of the uncertainty in this method arises from sampling errors of the gold-standard liver biopsy itself. Other sources of uncertainty are patient-specific differences in iron distribution, speciation, and hepatic water content. However, liver R2 assessment is highly reproducible, has been independently validated,[38] and is transferable across different types of MRI scanner. **Fig. 1** depicts work from the author's laboratory, independently confirming the initial R2-iron calibration. One specific liver R2 acquisition and analysis protocol, known as Ferriscan, has been approved by the Food and Drug Administration (FDA) as a clinical device.

Fig. 2 demonstrates the relationship between liver R2* and LIC. This relationship is linear and has confidence intervals of −46% to 44%; calibration was independently validated in a subsequent study.[39] Some confusion exists in the literature because calculated R2* values depend on the type of mathematical models used to fit the

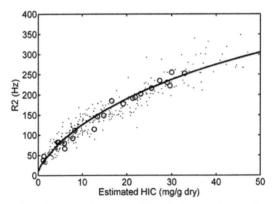

Fig. 1. Scattergram of liver R2 as a function of LIC by biopsy (*open circles*), or by liver R2* (*dots*).[38,69] Solid line represents the calibration curve originally published by St Pierre and colleagues,[37] not a fit to the data. Despite significant differences in scanner hardware, image acquisition, and post-processing techniques between the two laboratories, the overall agreement is excellent. (*From* Wood JC, Enriquez C, Ghugre N, et al. MRI R2 and R2* mapping accurately estimates hepatic iron concentration in transfusion-dependent thalassemia and sickle cell disease patients. Blood 2005;106:1460–5; with permission.)

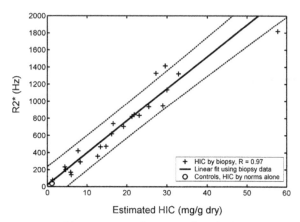

Estimated HIC (mg/g dry)

Fig. 2. (*Left*) Scattergram of liver R2* as a function of LIC by biopsy. Relationship is linear, with confidence intervals of −46% to 44%.[38] Calibration curve was independently validated.[39] (*From* Wood JC, Enriquez C, Ghugre N, et al. MRI R2 and R2* mapping accurately estimates hepatic iron concentration in transfusion-dependent thalassemia and sickle cell disease patients. Blood 2005;106:1460–5; with permission.)

MRI images. However, these biases are corrected when appropriate calibration curves are applied.[40]

Both R2 and R2* are suitable for LIC estimates in clinical practice if performed using validated acquisition and analysis protocols. R2 and R2* both are more accurate than liver biopsy for determining response to iron chelation therapy.[41] However, it is important to use the same technique when tracking patients over time.[42] Liver R2* is more robust than liver R2 for tracking chelation response on time scales 6 months or shorter, but R2 and R2* performances are equivalent for annual examinations. **Table 1** lists FDA-approved options for R2 and R2* analysis. Some centers, including the author's, use software developed in-house. All such tools require cross-validation with established techniques before clinical use. **Table 2** summarizes the advantages and disadvantages of both techniques.

Table 1	
FDA-approved imaging companies and analysis software	
Tool	**Description**
Ferriscan	A full-service imaging company that will guide tightly controlled image acquisition and provide an imaging report. A good option when local radiology expertise or interest is lacking. Billed as a charge per examination that must be passed to insurers or patients
CMR Tools Circle CMR42 Diagnosoft STAR Medis QMass	Stand-alone software that provides organ T2* measurements from suitably acquired images. Care must be taken to measure regions and truncate signal decay curves appropriately. Values are not reported in iron units, but calibration curves for liver and heart may be found in Refs.[49,70]; software can be licensed annually or purchased outright
ReportCard	MRI vendor-based T2* analysis packages. Some allow use of different fitting models. Cross-validation with other techniques is lacking for these tools at present. Software is generally purchased outright at the time of equipment acquisition

Table 2
Advantages and disadvantages of Ferriscan R2 versus R2* analysis

	Ferriscan R2	R2*
Speed	10 min per examination	<1 min
Validation	++++	++++
Reproducibility (%)	5–8	5–6
Quality control	Tight (by vendor)	Variable (by site)
Cost	$400 per examination	Variable. Approximately 10 min of technician time + software costs
Dynamic range (mg/g)	0–43	Variable, usually 0–35
Breathing artifact	Vulnerable to ghosting	Robust (breath-hold)
Metal/gas artifact	Robust	May affect usable region

MEASUREMENT OF NONHEPATIC IRON STORES

Although LIC is an excellent surrogate for total iron balance, it has limited ability to predict risk in extrahepatic organs. The endocrine glands and the heart develop pathologic iron overload exclusively through uptake of NTBI. The mechanism by which this uptake occurs is controversial, but L-type calcium channels have been implicated in some studies.[43] Regardless, it is possible for patients to develop progressive extrahepatic iron loading despite iron chelation keeping them in neutral total iron balance.[22,44] This situation is caused by the chelator having inadequate exposure to the chelatable iron pool, because it either does not enter the target organ or does not adequately suppress the circulating NTBI. **Fig. 3** shows the LIC of 26 chronically transfused patients who developed de novo cardiac iron load while under routine heart and liver iron surveillance at Children's Hospital Los Angeles, sorted by disease. All of the SCD patients had severe liver iron deposition before heart iron loading developed, whereas fewer than half of patients with other disease states

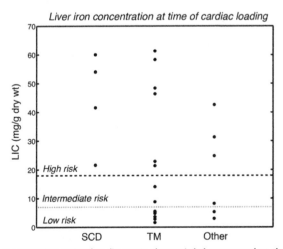

Fig. 3. Graph demonstrating LIC value (in mg/g dry weight) measured at the time heart iron became detectable. LIC values greater than 18 mg/g were considered high risk and LIC values between 7 mg/g and 18 mg/g assigned intermediate risk.

had LICs typically associated with cardiac iron. In fact, more than 40% of non-SCD patients had LICs of less than 7 mg/g, a level thought to be safe. Without routine cardiac surveillance, these patients would have ultimately developed endocrine and cardiac complications.[45]

Heart Iron

The first article linking MRI-detectable cardiac iron to patient symptoms was in 2001. At that time, the calibration curves for cardiac iron were not known and results were displayed using the relaxation time, T2* (**Fig. 4**A).[46] T2* values greater than 20 milliseconds are considered normal. All patients with thalassemia major having T2* values in this range had normal ejection fraction. As T2* declined to less than 20 milliseconds, there was an increasing prevalence of myocardial dysfunction, with a particularly high prevalence for T2* values less than 10 milliseconds.

Cardiac T2* was initially validated against cardiac iron concentration in animal models,[47] and later in 2 autopsy studies.[48,49] Cardiac T2* values can be converted to cardiac iron concentration using the following equation[49]:

$$\text{Cardiac iron concentration} = 45/(T2^*)^{1.22} \qquad (3)$$

Despite the availability of this equation, many articles continue to report results in T2* values because of physician familiarity with this metric.

The observation that many patients with cardiac iron loading had normal function puzzled initial investigators. However, MRI T2* is most sensitive to iron that is safely stored in hemosiderin deposits. Initially excess cardiac iron produces no ill effects, because ferritin-hemosiderin buffering systems in the myocyte are able to keep the toxic labile cellular iron levels low. However, with time or ongoing loading, a tipping point is reached and cardiac symptoms develop. This process was best demonstrated by a registry study[50] following 652 thalassemia patients from 21 centers in the United Kingdom (see **Fig. 4**B). The probability of developing congestive heart failure after 1 year was a powerful function of starting T2*, being less than 2% for a T2* value from 10 to 20 milliseconds and greater than 50% for a T2* of less than 6 milliseconds.

Based on these findings, a "stoplight" scheme is often applied to cardiac T2* values: values greater than 20 milliseconds are green, values between 10 and 20 milliseconds are yellow, and values less than 10 milliseconds are red. Many treatment paradigms use these designations, including a recent consensus paper from the American Heart Association.[51] A commentary summarizing the development of MRI as the gold standard for cardiac iron quantification may also be found in a different issue of the same journal.[52]

Pancreas Iron

Like the heart, the pancreas selectively takes up non–transferrin-bound iron species,[43] but it is a more sensitive predictor of long-term labile iron control.[53] **Fig. 5**A depicts the relationship between pancreas R2* and heart R2*. Note that there are regions where the pancreas is iron loaded with a clear heart, but the converse is never true. This finding reflects that pancreas is an early predictor of potential cardiac iron loading; a pancreas R2* of 100 Hz appears to represent a risk threshold.[54] Because the heart clears iron so slowly once it is loaded (half-life 14 months at maximal therapy), the author recommends responding to unfavorable trends in pancreatic iron rather than waiting for cardiac iron to accumulate.

Pancreas R2* values also predict endocrine function.[55] **Fig. 5**B demonstrates that the probability of having abnormal fasting glucose or oral glucose tolerance test

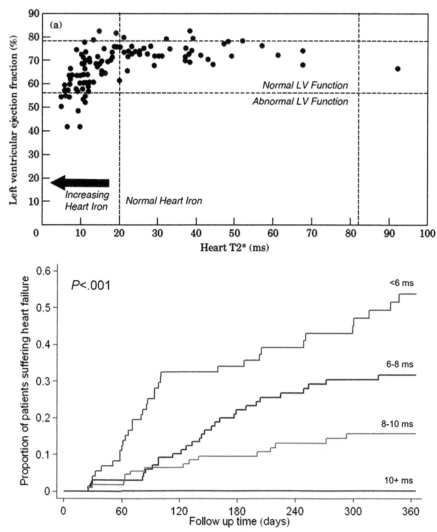

Fig. 4. (*Top*) Plot of left ventricular ejection fraction (in percent) versus heart T2* (in milliseconds). A T2* greater than 20 ms indicates that the heart is free of cardiac iron. Ejection fraction above 56% is considered normal. As heart iron increases (T2* declines) the prevalence of abnormal function increases.[46] (*Bottom*) Probability of developing clinical heart failure over a one year interval, based upon initial cardiac T2*. Cardiac T2* <6 ms was associated with nearly a 50% likelihood of developing heart failure over one year.[50] (*From* Anderson LJ, Holden S, Davis B, et al. Cardiovascular T2-star (T2*) magnetic resonance for the early diagnosis of myocardial iron overload. Eur Heart J 2001;22:2171–9; with permission. *From* Kirk P, Roughton M, Porter JB, et al. Cardiac T2* magnetic resonance for prediction of cardiac complications in thalassemia major. Circulation 2009;120:1961–8; with permission.)

(OGTT) increases as the pancreas and heart become iron loaded. While most patients with abnormal cardiac R2* also have overt diabetes, more than 50% of the patients with isolated pancreas iron overload manifested preclinical glucose dysregulation by OGTT.

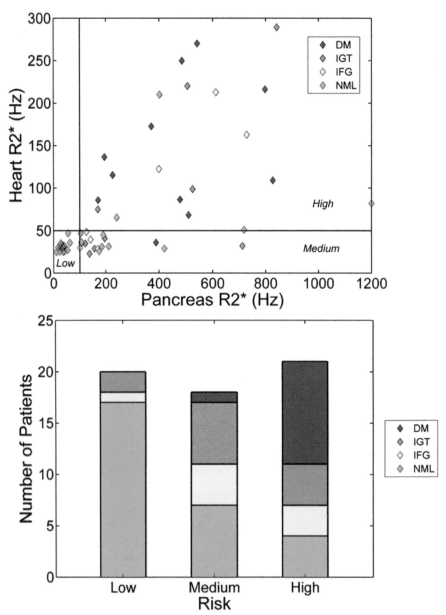

Fig. 5. (*Top*) Plot of heart R2* versus pancreas R2*.[55] Horizontal line at 50 Hz indicates the threshold of detectable heart iron. Vertical line at 100 Hz represents a risk threshold for pancreas R2*. Color of each diamond represents the outcome of an oral glucose tolerance test. Normal heart and normal pancreas represents low risk. Normal heart with abnormal pancreas represents medium risk. When both organs have iron overload, the patient is considered high risk. (*Bottom*) Results of OGTT test as a function of risk threshold.[55] DM, diabetes mellitus; IFG, impaired fasting glucose; IGT, impaired glucose tolerance; NML, normal glucose tolerance. (*From* Noetzli LJ, Mittelman SD, Watanabe RM, et al. Pancreatic iron and glucose dysregulation in thalassemia major. Am J Hematol 2012;87:155–60; with permission.)

Pituitary Iron

Hypogonadotropic hypogonadism remains the leading endocrinopathy in patients with thalassemia major, with a prevalence of approximately 50% in multicenter trials.[56,57] Although improved access to iron chelation is undoubtedly lowering this figure, monitoring of pituitary function cannot begin until puberty. Unfortunately, significant iron accumulation occurs during the first and second decades of life, producing irreversible gland destruction in early adulthood.[58] Pituitary iron accumulation is correlated with iron deposition in the liver, pancreas, and heart. However, heart deposition is late, and patients with increased cardiac iron are at high risk for hypogonadism.[58]

Because hypogonadism is only partially reversible with intensive chelation,[59] it is imperative to identify and treat preclinical pituitary iron deposition. Because the pituitary resides in a magnetically inhomogeneous environment (in the sella tursica), R2 imaging, rather than R2* imaging, is indicated. Imaging protocols for pituitary R2 and pituitary volume assessment are well established,[60] and age-specific and sex-specific normative values have been published. A Z_{vol} value of less than −2 indicates gland shrinkage below the 2.5th percentile and a Z_{R2} value greater than 2 indicates iron accumulation greater than the 97.5th percentile.

Risk thresholds for pituitary iron accumulation and gland shrinkage are shown in **Fig. 6**. Z_{R2} values less than −2.5 were associated with a high rate (88%) of hypogonadism. Moderate pituitary iron deposition ($2 < Z_{R2} < 5$) was not associated with clinical hypogonadism in this study, but biochemical hypogonadism was not assessed. By

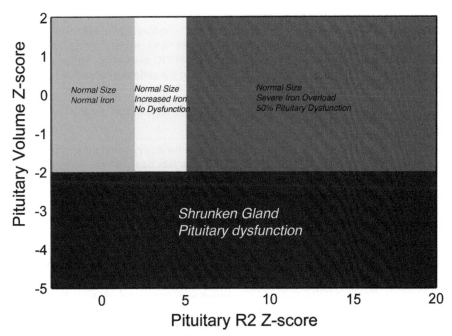

Fig. 6. Plot of pituitary size (Z-score) versus pituitary iron.[58,60] No pituitary dysfunction was observed when size and iron Z-scores were normal (*green*) or even when pituitary iron was moderately elevated (Z score 2 to 5, *yellow*).[58] However, hypogonadism was common (50%) in severe pituitary iron overload (Z >5, red zone) or when the pituitary gland was shrunken (Z score < −2.0).

contrast, 50% of the patients with severe pituitary iron deposition ($Z_{R2}>5$) were hypogonadal.

Standards for routine monitoring have not been established. The author recommends one scan between 7 and 10 years of age to identify patients with early-onset pituitary iron deposition. The second and early third decades are particularly dynamic from both a physiologic and emotional perspective. Monitoring is particularly important to identify and correct problems that may block the critical period for sexual and bone development.

The author has also used these techniques to probe intermittently transfused children with hypogonadism following bone marrow transplantation, head irradiation, or chemotherapy for acute myelogenous leukemia. Although results remain anecdotal, gland shrinkage also appears to have a high specificity for hypogonadism of for non–iron-mediated pituitary toxicities.

Kidney Iron

The most common source of iron deposition in the kidney is intravascular hemolysis. Decellularized hemoglobin (also known as plasma free hemoglobin) is filtered at the glomerulus, and actively taken up by megalin-cubulin receptors in the proximal and distal convoluted tubules.[61] This process creates a characteristic cortical darkening on MRI images, with complete sparing of the medulla.[62] Global kidney R2* values can reach 200 Hz, with cortical values of more than 1000 Hz, and are correlated with surrogates of hemolysis such as lactate dehydrogenase.[63] No correlations have been observed between kidney R2* and LIC in patients with hemolytic disease. The functional significance of renal iron deposits remains unproven, although no longitudinal studies have been performed to date.

Mild kidney R2* increases can also be observed in nonhemolytic anemias, but the iron deposition is not limited to the cortex. R2* values rarely exceed 60 Hz, and these mild elevations are typically only observed for severe LIC elevations. These changes may represent NTBI uptake and storage throughout the different renal cell types, as has been described on autopsy studies, but functional significance remains controversial.

Spleen Iron

Spleen R2* values are easy to measure using the same analysis and acquisition techniques as for the liver. No R2*-iron calibration curve has been directly validated, but indirect methods have been applied.[64] No functional significance for spleen iron accumulation has been determined to date.

IMPACT OF DISEASE STATE ON EXTRAHEPATIC IRON LOADING

Primary hemochromatosis and thalassemia intermedia syndromes are typically characterized by sparing of reticuloendothelial organs, such as the spleen, and only rarely lead to cardiac and endocrine involvement. Extrahepatic deposition does not typically occur until the fourth or fifth decade of life, usually after significant hepatic damage has already occurred.

By contrast, transfusional siderosis loads the bone marrow and reticuloendothelial system first, with liver parenchymal, endocrine, and cardiac iron loading later, in that order. However, the risk of extrahepatic iron loading varies considerably across different anemia subtypes. One of the strongest predictors is the rate of effective red cell production, reflected by the reticulocyte count. Red cell production requires transferrin-bound uptake into the bone marrow erythroid precursors, regenerating apo-transferrin and lowering transferrin saturation. Patients with Blackfan-Diamond anemia, which has the lowest transferrin utilization of any anemia, are particularly prone to cardiac and endocrine iron deposition. These patients may develop cardiac iron within just a first few years after starting transfusion therapy.[65,66] Patients with congenital dyserythropoietic anemia, thalassemia major, and aplastic anemia have intermediate risk, with cardiac iron typically occurring no less than 7 to 10 years after initiating transfusions when receiving appropriate transfusion and chelation therapy.[66] SCD patients represent the lowest risk category.[67] Many SCD patients retain high reticulocyte counts during chronic transfusion therapy, leading to lower transferrin saturations and circulating labile plasma iron levels.[64] Cardiac and endocrine iron deposition do occur in SCD patients, but later in life and at a slower rate than in chronically transfused thalassemia patients.[68]

RATIONAL MONITORING PRACTICES

MRI is a relatively expensive procedure, and care must be taken to use the resource wisely. However, monitoring costs are relatively modest in comparison with the cost of iron chelation medications and iron-mediated complications. **Fig. 7** is a flow chart outlining the author's clinical practice. Sometimes there is sufficient clinical knowledge to assign risk based purely on the patient's disease state, transfusion intensity, access to chelation, or MRI results from another institution. For example, low-risk patients include most SCD patients and transfusion-independent patients with iron overload. Low-risk patients only need MRI examination of the abdomen because a "clean" pancreas guarantees that the heart is free from significant iron deposition. The author defines an intermediate-risk patient as chronically transfused and having

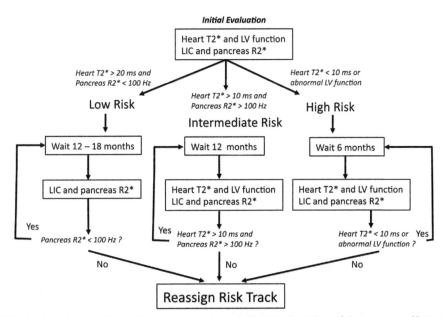

Fig. 7. Flow chart outlining the recommended monitoring algorithm. If there are insufficient clinical data to assign patients to a given monitoring track, all patients will undergo a baseline liver and heart iron examination for staging of clinical risk based on their cardiac T2* and pancreas R2* values. After each subsequent magnetic resonance imaging examination, patients are restratified, as necessary, to the appropriate monitoring track. LV, left ventricular.

sufficient transfusional exposure (usually >7 years for a patient with thalassemia major) to be at risk for cardiac iron overload. However, most patients receive heart and abdominal MRI examinations on the first visit, because their complete transfusion and chelation history is uncertain and because there can be genetic comodifiers of cardiac risk.

High-risk patients are defined as those whose cardiac T2* is less than 10 milliseconds. The author scans these patients at 6-month intervals for 3 reasons. First, it is important to monitor their left ventricular function. Even minor decreases in ventricular function are treated aggressively. Second, liver iron can change quickly during intensified therapy, and it is important to avoid overchelation. Lastly, regular scanning provides important feedback to the patients who often struggle with drug compliance.

AVAILABILITY OF MRI IRON ASSESSMENTS

With increased recognition of the utility of MRI in iron overload syndromes, the availability of individual medical centers to assess liver and cardiac iron is growing daily. Many radiology departments prefer to do the analyses themselves because there are financial and intellectual incentives to do so. However, quality control remains a significant problem in this regard unless the imaging centers take proper care to validate their acquisition techniques and their readers.

Some imaging centers are not interested in devoting the time necessary to maintain clinical competence in these metrics because imaging volume does not justify the financial overhead. In these situations, third-party solutions represent a "win-win" situation for radiology departments and practitioners interested in liver iron and cardiac T2* measurements.

Measurement of pancreatic R2* can be performed using the same techniques as for liver R2*. Fatty replacement of the gland complicates measurements in older subjects, and measurement variability is higher than for the other organs. Moreover, pancreas orientation is highly variable in splenectomized subjects, making measurement more challenging. Thus although pancreas R2* measurements are not universally obtained, they are gaining increasing acceptance. The author's laboratory is exploring novel methods to improve access to these techniques.

Pituitary R2, though also not universally performed, is a relatively easy and rapid measurement to obtain (4 minutes). Postprocessing is also more straightforward than for the liver, making it easy for most radiology departments to perform adequately. However, the specialty of iron overload is evolving so rapidly that a clinical niche for pituitary R2 assessments has not been firmly established. However, as more experimental data and clinical experience accumulate, pituitary R2 measurements are likely to increase in importance, especially in SCD and for survivors of pediatric malignancy.

SUMMARY

Serum ferritin and transferrin saturation remain valuable in tracking the therapeutic response to iron-removal therapies. However, these inexpensive techniques have many shortcomings that preclude using them safely as sole monitors for chelator efficacy. MRI has become the de facto gold standard for tracking iron levels in the body because it is accurate, reproducible, and well tolerated by patients, and can track iron levels in different organs of the body. The latter characteristic is important because the mechanisms and kinetics of iron uptake and clearance vary across somatic organs. The author's clinical practice is presented as a reference, but individual experiences will still be colored by local expertise as the technologies continue to mature and distribute.

REFERENCES

1. Cohen AR, Glimm E, Porter JB. Effect of transfusional iron intake on response to chelation therapy in beta-thalassemia major. Blood 2008;111:583–7.
2. Angelucci E, Brittenham GM, McLaren CE, et al. Hepatic iron concentration and total body iron stores in thalassemia major. N Engl J Med 2000;343: 327–31.
3. Brittenham GM, Cohen AR, McLaren CE, et al. Hepatic iron stores and plasma ferritin concentration in patients with sickle cell anemia and thalassemia major. Am J Hematol 1993;42:81–5.
4. Belhoul KM, Bakir ML, Saned MS, et al. Serum ferritin levels and endocrinopathy in medically treated patients with beta thalassemia major. Ann Hematol 2012;91: 1107–14.
5. Herbert V, Jayatilleke E, Shaw S, et al. Serum ferritin iron, a new test, measures human body iron stores unconfounded by inflammation. Stem Cells 1997;15: 291–6.
6. Kountouras D, Tsagarakis NJ, Fatourou E, et al. Liver disease in adult transfusion-dependent beta-thalassaemic patients: investigating the role of iron overload and chronic HCV infection. Liver Int 2013;33:420–7.
7. Chapman RW, Hussain MA, Gorman A, et al. Effect of ascorbic acid deficiency on serum ferritin concentration in patients with beta-thalassaemia major and iron overload. J Clin Pathol 1982;35:487–91.
8. Musallam KM, Cappellini MD, Wood JC, et al. Iron overload in non-transfusion-dependent thalassemia: a clinical perspective. Blood Rev 2012;26(Suppl 1): S16–9.
9. Puliyel M, Sposto R, Berdoukas VA, et al. Ferritin trends do not predict changes in total body iron in patients with transfusional iron overload. Am J Hematol 2014;89(4):391–4.
10. Crownover BK, Covey CJ. Hereditary hemochromatosis. Am Fam Physician 2013;87:183–90.
11. Wangruangsathit S, Hathirat P, Chuansumrit A, et al. The correlation of trans-ferrin saturation and ferritin in non-splenectomized thalassemic children. J Med Assoc Thai 1999;82(Suppl 1):S74–6.
12. Pootrakul P, Breuer W, Sametband M, et al. Labile plasma iron (LPI) as an indi-cator of chelatable plasma redox activity in iron-overloaded beta-thalassemia/HbE patients treated with an oral chelator. Blood 2004;104:1504–10.
13. Piga A, Longo F, Duca L, et al. High nontransferrin bound iron levels and heart disease in thalassemia major. Am J Hematol 2009;84:29–33.
14. Brittenham GM, Griffith PM, Nienhuis AW, et al. Efficacy of deferoxamine in pre-venting complications of iron overload in patients with thalassemia major. N Engl J Med 1994;331:567–73.
15. Angelucci E, Muretto P, Nicolucci A, et al. Effects of iron overload and hepatitis C virus positivity in determining progression of liver fibrosis in thalassemia following bone marrow transplantation. Blood 2002;100:17–21.
16. Jensen PD, Jensen FT, Christensen T, et al. Evaluation of myocardial iron by magnetic resonance imaging during iron chelation therapy with deferrioxamine: indication of close relation between myocardial iron content and chelatable iron pool. Blood 2003;101:4632–9.

17. Wood JC, Kang BP, Thompson A, et al. The effect of deferasirox on cardiac iron in thalassemia major: impact of total body iron stores. Blood 2010;116: 537–43.
18. Telfer PT, Prestcott E, Holden S, et al. Hepatic iron concentration combined with long-term monitoring of serum ferritin to predict complications of iron overload in thalassaemia major. Br J Haematol 2000;110:971–7.
19. Kanwar P, Kowdley KV. Diagnosis and treatment of hereditary hemochromatosis: an update. Expert Rev Gastroenterol Hepatol 2013;7:517–30.
20. Mancuso A. Hepatocellular carcinoma in thalassemia: a critical review. World J Hepatol 2010;2:171–4.
21. Mancuso A. Management of hepatocellular carcinoma: enlightening the gray zones. World J Hepatol 2013;5:302–10.
22. Noetzli LJ, Carson SM, Nord AS, et al. Longitudinal analysis of heart and liver iron in thalassemia major. Blood 2008;112:2973–8.
23. Wood JC, Glynos T, Thompson A, et al. Relationship between LPI, LIC, and cardiac response in a deferasirox monotherapy trial. Haematologica 2011;96(7): 1055–8.
24. Angelucci E, Baronciani D, Lucarelli G, et al. Needle liver biopsy in thalassaemia: analyses of diagnostic accuracy and safety in 1184 consecutive biopsies. Br J Haematol 1995;89:757–61.
25. Ambu R, Crisponi G, Sciot R, et al. Uneven hepatic iron and phosphorus distribution in beta-thalassemia. J Hepatol 1995;23:544–9.
26. Emond MJ, Bronner MP, Carlson TH, et al. Quantitative study of the variability of hepatic iron concentrations. Clin Chem 1999;45:340–6.
27. Villeneuve JP, Bilodeau M, Lepage R, et al. Variability in hepatic iron concentration measurement from needle-biopsy specimens. J Hepatol 1996;25:172–7.
28. Koh TS, Benson TH, Judson GJ. Trace element analysis of bovine liver: interlaboratory survey in Australia and New Zealand. J Assoc Off Anal Chem 1980;63: 809–13.
29. Butensky E, Fischer R, Hudes M, et al. Variability in hepatic iron concentration in percutaneous needle biopsy specimens from patients with transfusional hemosiderosis. Am J Clin Pathol 2005;123:146–52.
30. Goldberg HI, Cann CE, Moss AA, et al. Noninvasive quantitation of liver iron in dogs with hemochromatosis using dual-energy CT scanning. Invest Radiol 1982;17:375–80.
31. Wood JC, Mo A, Gera A, et al. Quantitative computed tomography assessment of transfusional iron overload. Br J Haematol 2011;153:780–5.
32. Nielsen P, Engelhardt R, Fischer R, et al. Noninvasive liver-iron quantification by computed tomography in iron-overloaded rats. Invest Radiol 1992;27:312–7.
33. Brittenham GM, Farrell DE, Harris JW, et al. Magnetic-susceptibility measurement of human iron stores. N Engl J Med 1982;307:1671–5.
34. Fischer R, Longo F, Nielsen P, et al. Monitoring long-term efficacy of iron chelation therapy by deferiprone and desferrioxamine in patients with beta-thalassaemia major: application of SQUID biomagnetic liver susceptometry. Br J Haematol 2003;121:938–48.
35. Gianesin B, Zefiro D, Musso M, et al. Measurement of liver iron overload: noninvasive calibration of MRI-R2* by magnetic iron detector susceptometer. Magn Reson Med 2012;67:1782–6.
36. Ghugre NR, Wood JC. Relaxivity-iron calibration in hepatic iron overload: probing underlying biophysical mechanisms using a Monte Carlo model. Magn Reson Med 2011;65:837–47.

37. St Pierre TG, Clark PR, Chua-Anusorn W, et al. Noninvasive measurement and imaging of liver iron concentrations using proton magnetic resonance. Blood 2005;105:855–61.
38. Wood JC, Enriquez C, Ghugre N, et al. MRI R2 and R2* mapping accurately estimates hepatic iron concentration in transfusion-dependent thalassemia and sickle cell disease patients. Blood 2005;106:1460–5.
39. Hankins JS, McCarville MB, Loeffler RB, et al. R2* magnetic resonance imaging of the liver in patients with iron overload. Blood 2009;113:4853–5.
40. Meloni A, Rienhoff HY Jr, Jones A, et al. The use of appropriate calibration curves corrects for systematic differences in liver R2* values measured using different software packages. Br J Haematol 2013;161:888–91.
41. Wood JC, Zhang P, Rienhoff H, et al. Liver MRI is better than biopsy for assessing total body iron balance: validation by simulation. Blood 2013;122:958.
42. Wood JC, Zhang P, Rienhoff H, et al. R2 and R2* are equally effective in evaluating Chronic response to iron chelation. Am J Hematol 2014;89(5):505–8.
43. Oudit GY, Trivieri MG, Khaper N, et al. Role of L-type Ca^{2+} channels in iron transport and iron-overload cardiomyopathy. J Mol Med 2006;84:349–64.
44. Anderson LJ, Westwood MA, Prescott E, et al. Development of thalassaemic iron overload cardiomyopathy despite low liver iron levels and meticulous compliance to desferrioxamine. Acta Haematol 2006;115:106–8.
45. Gabutti V, Piga A. Results of long-term iron-chelating therapy. Acta Haematol 1996;95:26–36.
46. Anderson LJ, Holden S, Davis B, et al. Cardiovascular T2-star (T2*) magnetic resonance for the early diagnosis of myocardial iron overload. Eur Heart J 2001;22:2171–9.
47. Wood JC, Otto-Duessel M, Aguilar M, et al. Cardiac iron determines cardiac T2*, T2, and T1 in the gerbil model of iron cardiomyopathy. Circulation 2005;112:535–43.
48. Ghugre NR, Enriquez CM, Gonzalez I, et al. MRI detects myocardial iron in the human heart. Magn Reson Med 2006;56:681–6.
49. Carpenter JP, He T, Kirk P, et al. On T2* magnetic resonance and cardiac iron. Circulation 2011;123(14):1519–28.
50. Kirk P, Roughton M, Porter JB, et al. Cardiac T2* magnetic resonance for prediction of cardiac complications in thalassemia major. Circulation 2009;120:1961–8.
51. Pennell DJ, Udelson JE, Arai AE, et al. Cardiovascular function and treatment in beta-thalassemia major: a consensus statement from the American Heart Association. Circulation 2013;128(3):281–308.
52. Wood JC. History and current impact of cardiac magnetic resonance imaging on the management of iron overload. Circulation 2009;120:1937–9.
53. Noetzli LJ, Coates TD, Wood JC. Pancreatic iron loading in chronically transfused sickle cell disease is lower than in thalassaemia major. Br J Haematol 2011;152:229–33.
54. Noetzli LJ, Papudesi J, Coates TD, et al. Pancreatic iron loading predicts cardiac iron loading in thalassemia major. Blood 2009;114:4021–6.
55. Noetzli LJ, Mittelman SD, Watanabe RM, et al. Pancreatic iron and glucose dysregulation in thalassemia major. Am J Hematol 2012;87:155–60.
56. Borgna-Pignatti C, Rugolotto S, De Stefano P, et al. Survival and complications in patients with thalassemia major treated with transfusion and deferoxamine. Haematologica 2004;89:1187–93.
57. Vogiatzi MG, Macklin EA, Trachtenberg FL, et al. Differences in the prevalence of growth, endocrine and vitamin D abnormalities among the various thalassaemia syndromes in North America. Br J Haematol 2009;146:546–56.

58. Noetzli LJ, Panigrahy A, Mittelman SD, et al. Pituitary iron and volume predict hypogonadism in transfusional iron overload. Am J Hematol 2012;87:167–71.

59. Farmaki K, Tzoumari I, Pappa C, et al. Normalisation of total body iron load with very intensive combined chelation reverses cardiac and endocrine complications of thalassaemia major. Br J Haematol 2010;148:466–75.

60. Noetzli LJ, Panigrahy A, Hyderi A, et al. Pituitary iron and volume imaging in healthy controls. AJNR Am J Neuroradiol 2012;33:259–65.

61. Gburek J, Birn H, Verroust PJ, et al. Renal uptake of myoglobin is mediated by the endocytic receptors megalin and cubilin. Am J Physiol Renal Physiol 2003;285:F451–8.

62. Solecki R, von Zglinicki T, Muller HM, et al. Iron overload of spleen, liver and kidney as a consequence of hemolytic anaemia. Exp Pathol 1983;23:227–35.

63. Schein A, Enriquez C, Coates TD, et al. Magnetic resonance detection of kidney iron deposition in sickle cell disease: a marker of chronic hemolysis. J Magn Reson Imaging 2008;28:698–704.

64. Brewer CJ, Coates TD, Wood JC. Spleen R2 and R2* in iron-overloaded patients with sickle cell disease and thalassemia major. J Magn Reson Imaging 2009;29:357–64.

65. Porter JB. Concepts and goals in the management of transfusional iron overload. Am J Hematol 2007;82:1136–9.

66. Wood JC, Origa R, Agus A, et al. Onset of cardiac iron loading in pediatric patients with thalassemia major. Haematologica 2008;93:917–20.

67. Wood JC, Tyszka JM, Ghugre N, et al. Myocardial iron loading in transfusion-dependent thalassemia and sickle-cell disease. Blood 2004;103:1934–6.

68. Meloni A, Puliyel M, Pepe A, et al. Cardiac iron overload in sickle cell anemia. Blood 2013;122:1013.

69. Wood JC. Magnetic resonance imaging measurement of iron overload. Curr Opin Hematol 2007;14:183–90.

70. Garbowski M, Carpenter JP, Smith G, et al. Calibration of improved T2* method for the estimation of liver iron concentration in transfusional iron overload. Blood 2009;114.

Index

Note: Page numbers of article titles are in **boldface** type.

Hematol Oncol Clin N Am 28 (2014) 765–773
http://dx.doi.org/10.1016/S0889-8588(14)00071-9
0889-8588/14/$ – see front matter © 2014 Elsevier Inc. All rights reserved.

hemonc.theclinics.com

Printed and bound by CPI Group (UK) Ltd, Croydon, CR0 4YY

03/10/2024

01040492-0012